Praise for the Author

"Every so often a teacher comes amongst us who has experienced firsthand that which they intend to convey to others.

For the entire thirteen years that I have known and sought Michèle's knowledge, she has always practiced her own advice and offered me and others practical solutions for a healthier outcome. The wisdom in this book is the accumulation of her life's dedication to the betterment of our health. Knowledge is our first step and "Digestive Solutions" offers the reader this through simple and effective strategies that will assist in the maintenance of our health and prevention of any serious ailments.

I commend this book to all those who aspire to achieving their optimal health ... this is a one-stop resource that will find its way beside your bed and on your kitchen bench."

Christopher Georgaki
CEO, Paradigm Systems International Pty. Ltd.

"Michèle Wolff has done a tremendous job in writing this inspiring and insightful book!

I would recommend this for both the health practitioner and someone wanting to improve their life by enhancing their digestive health.

This book contains so many valuable insights, clinical tips, and practical ideas for everybody. And wonderful recipe ideas to try too!

It is a fascinating, well-written book and certainly a valuable resource that I would recommend to my patients.

I would also definitely recommend this book to anyone wanting to improve their digestive health and in fact their overall health.
"Digestive Solutions" will inspire readers to take charge of their diet and lifestyle and do what it takes to make a difference to their lives.

Ann Vlass Naturopath; Research Scientist, Fertility expert,
Author, *"Master Your Body Signs"* educator (BAIA.com.au)

Praise for the Author

"An absolute must read for anyone who is interested in their digestive health! Michèle has put together her years of healthcare experience and passion for using food as medicine to make this fantastic guide to a happy gut. The information provided is from a true expert in the field of digestive wellbeing and each chapter provides a wealth of knowledge and answers many questions to those interested in this area. The simplicity of using food as medicine for health can be easily forgotten in today's lifestyle and this book provides motivation to eat new foods, new tastes and for people to start their own cooking adventures. This easy-to-read guide can be used by anyone and would also be a highly beneficial addition for a health practitioner or student's bookshelf. Brilliant work Michèle!"

Laura Elliott Naturopath

DETOX, DIGESTIVE AND WELLNESS SOLUTIONS

101 Proven Methods to Solve Your Tummy
and Other Health Problems Naturally

MICHÈLE WOLFF

BALBOA
PRESS

A DIVISION OF HAY HOUSE

Balboa Press books may be ordered through booksellers or by contacting:

Balboa Press
A Division of Hay House
1663 Liberty Drive
Bloomington, IN 47403
www.balboapress.com.au
1 (877) 407-4847

Print information available on the last page.

ISBN: 978-1-5043-0331-6 (sc)
ISBN: 978-1-5043-0332-3 (e)

Balboa Press rev. date: 11/30/2016

I dedicate this book to all of you who have the courage, persistence and commitment to take action in achieving your dreams of health by solving your digestive and other health problems. Sometimes the ride is bumpy but relish every moment of the experience as you propel yourself to greater health and achieve your desired destination.

Michèle Wolff

ACKNOWLEDGEMENTS

It has been an honour and privilege to write this book. As with any major project, there are a number of very special people who contributed to making this book happen. So, I'd like to take this opportunity to say "THANK YOU."

A special thank you to Deborah, Yveone, Mel, Ann, Julie, Sue, Sam, Chris and Adam for your willingness to share your insights, your time and encouragement.

Next, a huge thanks to my staff, past and present; Laura and Kathleen (thank you both for your valuable help with the book layout), Rochelle, Sarah, Vanessa, Nicole, Claire, Nadia, Esther, Gen, Nina, Susan and Helen, your talents and care are much appreciated, you're truly amazing people!

To all of my clients, from who I have learnt so much.

A special thank you to my Mum & Dad and siblings Tim, Paul, Suzie, Christianne, Andrew and Marie-Francoise, I'm blessed with the richness and support of a big family.

To Tony for his brilliant work and patience in all the ongoing changes...thanks for your flexibility! I am truly grateful for your understanding in my continuous journey to success and for keeping up with me during the challenging moments. You're simply one-of-a-kind.

A huge thank you to Darren Stephens, my mentor and publisher at Global Publishing Group and to their awesome team, for your dedication and commitment to the book's success.

CONTENTS

Free Bonus Gift

Valued at $197 but yours FREE!

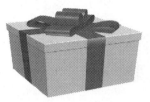

Claim your Free Bonus Gift by going to
www.colonicsandbowelhealth.com

You'll discover in these powerful videos
and health reports....

Simple yet effective techniques you can
apply to improve digestive health
What influences digestive health?
Why detox for optimum health?
Plus much much more.

Claim your free gift by going to
www.colonicsandbowelhealth.com

FOREWORD

As a doctor in both conventional and complementary medicine, I found Digestive Solutions very educational and entertaining.

Diseases of the digestive system affect millions of people and have a great impact on individuals and the health system of every country around the world. Digestive Solutions offers a wealth of knowledge and practical advice for resolving gut problems.

Digestive Solutions provides significant and valuable information on holistic health, such as diet and lifestyle, that is not usually given in modern medicine. It will help anyone who wants to improve their digestive and overall health. It's an invaluable resource for health professionals.

Professor Ian Brighthope

INTRODUCTION

The information offered in this book can be life changing. Many diseases can be greatly improved and often healed by maintaining and restoring a healthy digestive system. Treatment at the digestive level addresses many symptoms, root causes and inflammatory processes of illness. Improving digestion also reduces reactivity to foods which can play havoc with your health.

Often in your younger days you can eat what you want without significant signals that something is going wrong. It is best to avoid possible outcomes and treat yourself well now. Some of you may be more sensitive and have an assortment of digestive problems which need to be resolved; this book offers you a wealth of knowledge.

All adults want to know what it's like to feel vibrant and alive and all parents want to know the joys of raising a healthy child. This book will help you heal a range of tummy problems and increase your overall well-being. The emotional distress that people go through because of common digestive complaints can be avoided by eating the right foods and eliminating the harmful ones. Being responsible for what we eat can be a challenge and there are many practical solutions offered in this book. It will guide you to a nutritionally balanced and healing diet. You will be encouraged to nurture yourself to wellness and feel empowered to make good decisions for yourself.

The addition of over 50,000 additives, preservatives and colours to food is not acceptable and is causing harm. Allergies often come from a sick digestive system and other factors like pesticides and poor quality food. Diet has an extraordinary impact both negatively and positively and change is needed amongst communities, to eat well and think about their food choices. What you eat can affect the genetics of 3 generations and when enough people make positive food choices the food industry will change. Enjoy the healing path and positively enriching your life. You are what you eat, absorb and assimilate. I encourage you to use the valuable information in the resource section at the back.

"You as a food buyer, have the distinct privilege of proactively participating in shaping the world your children will inherit."

Joel Salatin

CHAPTER 1

How your digestive system works
A machine with many parts.

"All disease starts in the gut."

Hippocrates
(460 B.C. - 377 B.C.)

CHAPTER 1
How your digestive system works.
A machine with many parts.

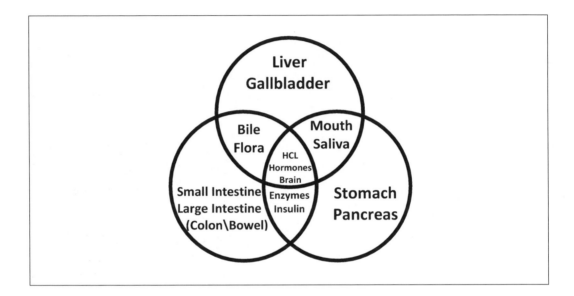

So that you can understand what's wrong with you and how to correct your health, it's important to know your body and how your digestive system works. Once you understand the digestive system and all its parts, it will make you more conscious about what you eat, your lifestyle and your stress levels. You will get to know how these things affect the tubes in your tummy. You may start to think twice about tins and packets of processed food.

When I was 18 years old I went to live with an Indonesian family in Bali for a short time. What amazed me was they had never seen a packet or tin of processed food, not even a can of soft drink. The mother went to the market nearly every day to buy fresh food and there was no fridge or freezer for storage. There was a well in the small back yard for water and camping type stoves for cooking. Yet these people ate the finest food, not because they could but because that was all that was available. Each meal consisted of fresh vegetables, rice, fresh herbs and meat or fish.

They were poor but vital, youthful and healthy. Their digestive system was not overloaded with toxins and they didn't have problems with elimination; they had a relaxed lifestyle. Even the teenagers were healthy as there were no fast food venues; alcohol wasn't part of the culture as it was just too expensive. The only thing some of them did now and then was to buy cigarettes from street stalls but they could only afford to buy 2 at a time for a treat. It was all so different from a western teenage lifestyle.

A more luxurious life in the west has bought with it chemicals, toxins and unhealthy attitudes and it's not always easy to step away from what's around you.

If you can make a difference to your digestion at a young age or give your kids a healthy start then there's a lot less unravelling to do when you are older. However, digestive woes can be completely reversed if you're prepared to help yourself. By working your way through this book and following the advice within you will start to see big shifts and improvements in your health. The digestive system is a long complex system with many parts. If you look after your nutrition and eliminate wastes effectively you are on your way to great health. You are what you

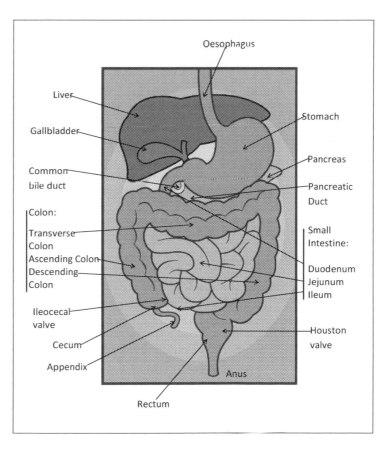

eat, assimilate and eliminate. The problem is that most of us either have inadequate nutrition to feed our cells effectively or we are not getting rid of our waste products sufficiently.

So what's underneath all that soft flesh on your tummy and how does it all work?

The digestive system is the most important system in your body as it feeds and nourishes the rest of your body and acts as a rubbish dump to carry away debris. The digestive system is also known as the gastrointestinal system. It consists of hollow tubes and supportive digestive organs that connect alongside it to help your body break down food. This includes the mouth, oesophagus which connects to the throat and the stomach, the stomach, liver, intestines, gall bladder and pancreas.

There are several words for the digestive system

Gastrointestinal and gut refer to the whole digestive tract. Intestines= large intestines= colon= bowel. Small intestines= small bowel. The stomach sits above the intestines.

The gut usually means the stomach and intestine but can refer to either.

Stools= faeces=poo!

The bowel

There are two parts to the intestines known as the colon/large intestine/bowel and small intestine or the variables above.

The small intestine joins the stomach and consists of the duodenum, jejunum and ileum. It then joins the large intestine via a valve called the ileocecal valve and can be a massive 7 metres long but half the width of the large intestine.

The large intestine/colon consists of the cecum, appendix, ascending colon, transverse colon, descending colon, sigmoid colon, houston valve, rectum and anus and is 1.5 metres long. In total the intestines are the width of a tennis court and when spread out cover the size of a double tennis court!

Throughout the digestive tract is a lining called the mucosa. In the mouth, stomach and small intestine your mucosa has small glands that produce juices to help digest food. The intestines have a layer of smooth muscle that with the juices helps break down your food and move it along so it can be absorbed and excreted.

Valves

There are two important valves, the ileocecal valve which joins the small and large intestine near the cecum. The other one, the houston valve, is in the rectum above the anus. It consists of 3 large folds that support the weight of faecal matter and prevent its urging toward the anus, which would produce a strong urge to defecate. Both of these can be damaged though constipation, inflammation stress and other means.

Digestive Organs

Two really important organs for digestion are the liver and pancreas. They produce essential juices for digestion. Between meals, the gall bladder stores juices from the liver and are known as bile. When the small intestine needs these juices the gall bladder squirts bile through ducts into the small intestine. Bile is green in colour and it is what makes the final colour of your stools (poo) brown. Bile is particularly needed to break down fat and helps dissolve it; rather like using a cleaning product to get grease off your oven. After fat is dissolved it is then digested by enzymes (an enzyme is a substance that speeds up chemical reactions in the body) from the pancreas and lining of the small intestine. Of course you also need a good blood supply and healthy functioning nerves to keep your digestive system healthy.

What happens when you eat?

Firstly your **saliva** produces enzymes that start breaking down food in your mouth; so chewing is very important. You don't want to swallow big chunks of food as it puts a lot of strain on the stomach and makes it difficult to break down your food to a soup-like substance called chyme.

There was a case of people stranded on an island with nothing to eat but poisonous berries. They ate the berries thinking they were healthy. Only one survived and it happened that this man had savoured them for so long in his mouth with lots of chewing that the saliva actually neutralised the poison.

The **stomach** lining produces stomach acid called Hydrochloric acid (HCl). The stomach has a thick mucus layer to stop the acid digesting the lining of the stomach itself and HCl is powerful at breaking down food and killing unfriendly microbes like parasites; then it empties into the small intestine. As you age, HCl production declines affecting your absorption of minerals and your first line of defence against all sorts of nasty bugs. If you eat lots of sugar it stops you from producing the hormone called gastrin that helps produce HCl. With low HCl you become more susceptible to inflammation and sugars from carbohydrates can ferment into unfriendly bacteria in the large intestine. Usually, food stays in the stomach between 1 and 5 hours. Common symptoms of low HCl include: burning from putrefaction of food (people often think this is too much acid but this is rare), bloating shortly after a meal especially with protein, bad breath, weak nails, iron deficiency, parasites, yeast infections and allergies. It is important to get a correct diagnosis. If you take 2 tablespoons of apple cider vinegar after a meal in ¼ cup of water and you feel better you are likely to have an HCl deficiency. Bitter foods, like bitter green leafy vegetables, watercress and bitter melon help the stomach cells produce more HCL; ginger, green tea and lemon can also help.

There are a few things that affect the stomach emptying into the **small intestine** which includes the types of foods eaten and the amount of muscle action needed to empty the contents of the stomach into the small intestine. Fat, for example, stays in the stomach the longest (fat is a rich source of energy and is stored in different parts of the body), then protein (this is necessary for building and repairing tissues and cells) and carbohydrates (glucose is the end product of carbohydrate digestion and is stored in the liver to provide energy for the body) take the least amount of time. Other vital parts of food that are absorbed in the small intestine are minerals including calcium, magnesium, sodium, potassium, iron, zinc, selenium, manganese, chromium, phosphorus, molybdenum and micro minerals. Vitamins are also absorbed, including the water soluble vitamins all B's and C (where excess is not stored but passed out in urine) and fat soluble vitamins A,D,E and K that are stored in the liver and fat.

When you eat food it has to be changed into smaller particles so that nutrition can be absorbed and taken around your blood and into the cells of your body to give you health and vitality. Your small intestine absorbs most of your nutrition. Your small intestine contains juices which mix with bile from the gall bladder and enzymes and digestive juices from the pancreas to dissolve your food further. These particles become small enough to be absorbed through the walls of the small intestine and the nutrients are then transported around the body. A lack of digestive enzymes can cause: bloating 1-2 hours after a meal especially with carbohydrates, food particles visible in the stool, fatty stools, allergies, hair loss, gas and diarrhoea. It is important to get an accurate diagnosis. Bromelain in pineapple and papain in pawpaw provide enzymes for digestion. The mucosa of the small intestine contains many folds with finger like projections called villi which are covered with microvilli. This gives a large surface area through which nutrients can be absorbed into the bloodstream.

The part of food that is not fully digested (which includes fibre and old cells that are shed from the mucosa wall) moves as waste from the small intestine to the large intestine through the ileocecal valve and takes about 8 hours.

The large intestine (bowel, colon) is the last part of the digestive system. Waste matter passes to the beginning of the large intestine, the caecum. Water is needed to help food particles move along the intestine and stop it drying out. The appendix is near the caecum and has lymphatic cells to carry away toxins which are important for immunity. These lymphatic cells are most active when you are a child and teenager. Appendicitis is the result of a blockage that traps infectious material in the appendix.

Waste material moves up the ascending colon and the colon's function is to move waste and absorb water and any remaining absorbable nutrients which are created by the colonic bacteria - such as vitamin K and the B vitamins. Important flora helps the absorption of some nutrients and aids in keeping bad bugs away. There are over 700 different types of good flora in the large and small intestine weighing about 2 kg. Waste material that has no purpose in the body moves across the transverse colon and down the descending colon to the rectum and is evacuated as faeces via the anus. If you have a prolapsed transverse colon, going on a slant board for 20 minutes a day and consuming silica rich foods is helpful as is colonic hydrotherapy. The large intestine is over 1.5 metres long and a lot wider than the small intestine. It has muscles with folds that help it move in a wave like action called peristalsis.

The large intestine takes about 16 hours to finish the digestion of food. Lack of magnesium can cause spasms in the large intestine. Colic, diarrhoea and pain can occur from irritation of the bowel wall. Often if there is pain, it comes a few hours after eating. There is a lot more on food in chapters 11 and 12.

Foods that help the large intestine

Magnesium rich foods help with spasms and cramps, like buckwheat, brown rice, nuts and seeds.

Protein and silica rich foods help strengthen the connective tissue on the bowel wall. Eggs, fish, beans, legumes, whole grains, horsetail tea, vegetables and fruits help.

Liquorice and turmeric help with inflammation.

Fermented foods help flora.

Foods that help the stomach, small intestine and pancreas

Apple cider vinegar, lemon juice, turmeric, coriander, fennel, liquorice, cardamom and fermented foods.

Foods to avoid

Gluten, dairy, peanuts, sugar, junk food and alcohol.

Digestion controlled by hormones

There are various hormones that help control the function of the digestive system. These hormones are produced and released by the cells in the mucosa of the stomach and small intestine. They move into the blood vessels of the digestive system then travel back to the heart which pumps them back into the digestive system where they stimulate the digestive juices and cause the digestive organs to move.

There are 3 main hormones that control digestion

Gastrin causes the stomach to produce acid to dissolve food and helps cell growth in the lining of the stomach, small and large intestines.

Secretin causes the pancreas to produce a juice that contains bicarbonate and neutralises acid contents from the stomach as they go into the small intestine. Secretin also causes the stomach to produce pepsin which is an enzyme that digests protein and it stimulates the liver to produce bile.

Cholecystokinin (CCK) causes the pancreas to produce enzymes in pancreatic juice, promotes cell growth in the pancreas and stimulates the gall bladder to empty.

Other hormones

Ghrelin is produced when the stomach is empty, so it stimulates appetite.

Peptide YY is produced in the digestive tract to tell you when you are full so it inhibits appetite.

Insulin is considered a hormone and is produced by your pancreas in response to eating sugars and carbohydrates. It causes cells in the liver, skeletal muscles and fat tissue to take up glucose (sugars are broken down to this) from the blood. In the liver and skeletal muscles, glucose is stored as glycogen which can be used as an energy source when needed. Insulin is provided to remove excess glucose from the blood, which otherwise would be toxic. Eating sugar and white flour and drinking alcohol and soft drinks regularly, causes the pancreas to burn out and the control of insulin fails leading to insulin resistance and diabetes. So many people have an overworked pancreas that is exhausted beyond belief.

The liver has a major impact on your digestive function. As your body is exposed to a considerable variety of toxins, good functioning of the liver is necessary for good health. The liver is the body's main detoxifying organ. The liver neutralises toxic substances into relatively non toxic molecules that can be excreted. The water soluble molecules are excreted in urine via the kidneys and fat soluble molecules are transformed and excreted through the bile via the gall bladder and through faeces in the bowel. If you are overloaded with toxins, low in nutrients or your bowel and other organs are working inefficiently, then there may be considerable toxic stress known as free radical production and oxidation. The toxins may accumulate which may cause damage to your liver and other organs.

As mentioned before the liver and gall bladder are also vital in digestion and work together with the small intestine to digest fats.

Foods that help the liver

- Bitter green leafy vegetables including rocket, endives, kale and bitter melon.

- Dandelion root tea.

- Lemon juice.

Foods to avoid

- Excess fat

- Poor quality fats

- Sugar

- Excess salt

- Fast foods

- Refined food

- Caffeine

- Alcohol

Water is very important.

Gut-associated lymphoid tissue and immunity

About 70% of the immune system is located in the gut as this is where protection is needed most from the onslaught of daily toxins. The immune system attacks these toxins or foreign particles. Stomach acid and a healthy mucosa wall in the gut help get rid of harmful substances. Food and water are the most common sources of toxic invasion so the gut needs the most immune protection. The gut is approximately 200 times the area of the skin and is the main entry site for environmental toxins. The inflammatory response is the next line of defence. It is vital for our survival but when it becomes chronic it can lead to chronic disease like auto immune disease.

When immunity is down and inflammation is up there can be an inability to respond to parasitic invasion. When there is damage to the gut there is more strain on the liver as anything that passes through the gut wall goes straight to the liver via the portal vein. As you heal your gut taking pressure off the liver is also important.

Now this may all seem a bit complicated but it's just to show you the detail of the immunity in the bowel and impress upon you how important it is.

The digestive tract's immune system is often referred to as **gut-associated lymphoid tissue (GALT)** and works to protect the body from invasion.

In fact, the intestine possesses the largest mass of lymphoid tissue in the human body. The GALT is made up of several types of lymphoid tissue that store immune cells. These cells include white cells called macrophages within the lining of the bowel. Within the sub-mucosa lining of the bowel are immune cells known as T helper cells. They both carry out attacks and defend against unfriendly substances, a bit like a 'pacman' that looks for debris and gobbles it up.

Good gut flora has a big impact on the positive activity of GALT and immunity. A healthy gut makes a healthy person.

Lymphoid tissue in the gut helps carry away toxins and boosts immunity

GALT includes:

- Appendix.

- Numerous solitary lymphoid follicles.

- Peyer's patches which are collections of lymphoid tissue in the lowest part of the small intestine, the ileum. They help immunity and are on the lookout for invading particles.

The main Drivers of immune disease are:

- Diet

- Lack of Exercise

- Obesity

- Stress

- Toxicity

- Hormonal Metabolism

- Genetic Factors

All of these can contribute to inflammation and the most important is diet.

Foods that can cause inflammation include: refined starches, sugar, junk food, poor fats, lack of antioxidants, coffee, soft drinks and energy drinks. Gluten found in barley, rye, oats and wheat can cause inflammation for many people and the sensitivity in its severe form results in coeliac disease.

Foods that help are: fibre foods, vegetables, turmeric and omega 3 foods, like fish and flaxseed oil. Diet induced inflammation underlies most chronic diseases. It's not always the food itself but additives within the food.

Food intolerance/allergy can lead to autoimmune (when the body attacks its own tissues, resulting in inflammation) diseases such as:

- Diabetes

- Dermatitis

- Lupus

- Microscopic Colitis

- Psoriasis

- Rheumatoid Arthritis

- Thyroid Disease

From an anatomical perspective, the key to a good digestion is:

Good amounts of HCl in the stomach, a healthy liver for detoxifying and producing adequate amounts of bile to be released by the gall bladder, a healthy pancreas to release digestive enzymes and insulin, effective elimination through the intestines and a healthy intestinal wall that promotes immunity and positive micro-organisms. The digestive tract has more nerve endings than any other system in the body and this is important for motility and the gut/brain connection.

How digestive organs can behave

The following chart explains the digestive system and symptoms of imbalance. With the organ times if you wake up at the times shown or have discomfort at these times it can often be related to a corresponding organ. For example, eating a food that is difficult to digest may have you waking up between 1 and 3a.m. if it taxes your liver or at 5 and 7a.m. if it taxes your large intestine. It's usually related to food or drink consumed the day before but can relate to chronic problems.

Organ	Function	Acute Symptoms	Chronic Symptoms
Stomach **Chinese clock** **time 7 - 9 am.** **Emotion** **Anxiety,** **hypersensitivity**	Secretes gastric enzymes and hydrochloric acid. Secretes intrinsic factor for B12 absorption and protective mucus. Main location for protein digestion. Mixes food and breaks it down.	Burping with strong offensive smell. Hunger pains. Pain before and between meals. Excessive mucus production. Poor digestion due to tight muscles. Heartburn. Upper abdominal pain. Vomiting.	Tiredness after a meal. Slow digestion. Gas. Bloating after protein. Bad breath. Immediate pain after eating. Lack of mucus leading to ulcers. Lack of muscle tone/ poor digestion. Lack of B12 absorption.

Organ	Function	Acute Symptoms	Chronic Symptoms
Pancreas **Chinese clock** **time 9 - 11 am.** **Emotion** **Pensive,** **obsessive,** **regretful, worry**	Secretes pancreatic enzymes and juices into the small intestine to break down protein, fats and carbohydrates. Secretes buffer solution bicarbonate to alkalise.	Blood sugar issues. Diabetes. Indigestion caused by excessive production of enzymes and bicarbonate affecting digestive hormones and causing quick release into the intestines. Overly alkaline blood.	Sweet cravings. Bloating after carbohydrates and or protein. Allergies. Poor absorption. Smelly stools. Duodenal ulcer. Acidity from lack of bicarbonate. Blood sugar issues. Diabetes. Fatigue.
Liver **Chinese clock** **time 1 - 3 am.** **Emotion Anger/** **frustration**	Makes bile for the small intestine to break down and absorb fat. Other functions; produces substances for immunity and blood thinning. Gets rid of old red blood cells and bacteria. Detoxifies body acids and metabolic wastes. Stores and releases sugar into the blood by storing glucose. Stores vitamins A, D, E and K, along with copper, iron and poisons in the body.	Nausea, burping, headaches. Temperature up at night and low in the morning. Hepatitis. Fatty deposits. Overweight. Acidity of blood/high urea content. Metals can concentrate in the liver. Jaundice. Skin pigmentation. Diarrhoea. Hot sweats and cold chills.	Poor healing. Lowered immunity. Cold. Weight loss and gain. Poor fat absorption. Pale stools. Low blood sugar. Fatigue. Faintness. Hunger pangs. Broken capillaries/bruising. Low libido. Constipation. Anaemia. Psoriasis. Acne. Eczema.

Gall Bladder Chinese clock time 11 pm.- 1 am. Emotion Resentment/ decision making	Stores bile and releases it into the small intestine for fat digestion. Removes sodium from bile and pumps it back to the blood plasma. Removes water from bile to increase the concentration of bile salts.	Pain under right shoulder. Right upper abdominal pain. Nausea. Can't sit still. Heart burn. Jaundice. Watery stools.	Undigested fats in stools. Gallstones. Loss of appetite. Constipation.
Organ	**Function**	**Acute Symptoms**	**Chronic Symptoms**
Small Intestine Chinese clock time 1 - 3 pm. Emotion Power of discernment and good judgement	Most digestion and absorption of nutrients occurs here.	Inflammatory pain, pain from obstruction and inflammatory bowel disease. Bloating ½ an hour or more after a meal - poor enzymes. Allergic symptoms.	Pain and bloating from parasites, viruses, fungus. Weakness and poor absorption from diseases like coeliac, anorexia and bulimia.
Large Intestine Chinese clock time 5 – 7 am. Emotion Tension, dwelling in the past, not going with the flow	It takes about 16 hours to finish the digestion of food. Absorbs water and vitamins made by colonic bacteria. Eliminates waste.	Pain from Crohn's disease, colitis and diverticulitis. Constipation. Diarrhoea. Bleeding from haemorrhoids, polyps or cancer.	Chronic constipation, diarrhoea and bloating. Pain from spasms and inflammation. Poor flora and a lack of minerals can lead to these problems.

Digestive illnesses

The number 1 selling drug in America is Nexium for gastrointestinal disorders, Remicade for Crohn's disease is in the top 8, Zantac is also high on the list which is used for digestive problems, including prevention of ulcers and for reflux and laxatives are used daily; an alarming $500 is spent per man, woman and child per year on laxatives! Isn't this telling us it's high time to change our dietary and lifestyle habits?

Appendicitis is a medical emergency and requires an operation. Usually there is pain in the right lower abdomen, then vomiting and fever. I have known a rumbling appendix resolved by colonic hydrotherapy (closed method) and flaxseed tea and slippery elm also help. (Ch. 12)

Bad breath can be due to tooth and gum problems, post nasal drip, sinusitis, smoking, stomach problems like reflux, kidney failure (rare) and certain foods like garlic. A clean diet with no white flour or sugar, adequate water and herbs like thyme, cinnamon and cloves can help.

Bleeding needs to be investigated. Small amounts of fresh blood often mean haemorrhoids or fissures. Black stools can indicate bleeding higher up in the colon. Larger amounts of fresh blood can occur in ulcerative colitis and tumours.

Bloating can be caused by weak digestion (pancreas and liver are involved), lack of digestive juices, parasites, fungus, food intolerances, fluid retention, small intestine bacterial overgrowth, gas and cancer.

Bowel cancer

80% of bowel cancers are found in two places, the caecum area and the sigmoid rectal area. Bowel cancers seem to form where faecal contents sit and stagnate. This builds up toxins from rotting waste and damages the cells of the bowel. A lack of positive nutrients to mop up the toxins is also a causative factor. Bowel cancer is on the increase and cancer is the leading cause of death in children under 15 years old in Australia. Alarmingly, cancer is the leading cause of death in adults in Australia according to the Australian Institute of Health. Not surprisingly, the physicians committee for responsible medicine shows that diet is the greatest single factor in the epidemic of cancer. Yet how many doctors tell you to see an expert in diet therapy? The institute of cancer research shows that food additives, chemicals preservatives, artificial sweeteners, hydrogenated oils, MSG, artificial colours, sodium benzoate, potassium benzoate and BHA and BHT in snack foods are all potentially carcinogenic. On top of that corn syrup, dried fruit, sodium sulphite in wine and canned olives can be carcinogenic and cause allergies and heart palpitations. So think about what your gut has to cope with and eliminate these nasties. It's time to eat whole fresh foods; after all, eating a tasty apple is easier to eat than artificial snack foods.

The Institute of Cancer Research in America recommends 5-8 servings of fruit and vegetables daily, 6-8 glasses of water daily and walking for 30-40 minutes daily to help prevent cancer. Garlic, onions and broccoli are protective against cancer. You can imagine why bowel cancer develops especially when these toxins get slowed down by constipation.

Candida (Ch.5)

Coeliac - there are often allergies and damage to the gut wall. Avoid all gluten, including: barley, rye, oats, spelt and wheat. Leaky gut is common. Slippery elm, pectin from apples, guar gum, pumpkin seeds for zinc and probiotic foods listed in Ch.9 help.

Colitis/inflammatory bowel disease/(ulcerative colitis is a more severe form of colitis) involves inflammation of the intestinal lining. It often occurs not only with a poor diet but also when there are inflammatory emotions, in other words a lot of stress. It can follow a bowel infection or nasty parasites. A low reactive diet avoiding wheat, dairy, sugar and tomatoes is helpful as is addressing enzymes, flora, reducing inflammation with herbs like turmeric, liquorice and chamomile tea. Help the gut lining with slippery elm and boost immunity with vegetables and garlic. See raw cabbage juice (Ch.11). The same herbs mentioned in Crohn's are helpful as well as kefir, yoghurt and aloe vera.

Constipation (Ch.6)

Crohn's is known as an autoimmune disease where the bowel attacks itself. This usually starts with stress and a leaky gut which I talk about later. It is very debilitating with a lot of inflammation. A simple unprocessed diet is essential and herbs you can use in your cooking include turmeric and coriander. Aloe vera, ginger, chamomile, liquorice, garlic and oily fish are beneficial. Follow advice for colitis.

Diarrhoea can be caused by a bug, off food, food intolerances, malabsorption, viruses, drug reactions, functional bowel disorders and bowel diseases like Crohn's. Mild diarrhoea is best left alone as it's natural for your body to get rid of toxins but keep well hydrated. If it is severe or lasts more than 3 days, eat cooked white rice, drink coconut water and eat grated apple skin but allow it to go brown first.

Diverticulitis - itis at the end of a word means inflammation and diverticula are outpouching sacs on the bowel wall. They usually occur in the large intestine but can become inflamed and bleed and this is diverticulitis. Chronic pressure, constipation and a poor diet can contribute to this as well as a lack of certain nutrients like silica which helps keep the bowel wall strong.

It is best to eat the fibre and anti-inflammatory foods mentioned in chapter 11 and to be careful with eating seeds or nuts which can get stuck in the pouch and cause it to become inflamed.

Dysbiosis is a lack of good intestinal flora that allows bad bacteria to grow. It can cause many abdominal symptoms and can be diagnosed with a simple test by your naturopath.

Fissure is a split in the anal wall. It can be very painful and is usually caused by diarrhoea, constipation, inflammation or a poor diet. Wheat grass works wonders for fissures. Lavender oil helps pain and stimulates healing. Foods high in bioflavonoids and silica help healing e.g. the pith of citrus fruits and buckwheat, nettle leaf and horsetail tea.

Gas/flatulence/wind/farting are all the same thing. There can be several causes of gas; parasites and fungus, intolerances and allergies to certain foods including fructose and lactose intolerance and an imbalance of good intestinal flora or a lack of it. Foods containing oligosaccharides like beans and lentils can cause gas as well as foods containing sulphur, like garlic and onions.

Haemorrhoids are caused by pressure on the rectum causing veins to enlarge, bulge and sometimes bleed. They can occur during pregnancy or birth, by sitting for long periods, be a result of chronic constipation and a lack of certain nutrients like bioflavonoids and silica which can be found in buckwheat and the pith (white lining) of citrus fruit.

Helicobacter Pylori is bacteria in the stomach which can cause chronic inflammation and lead to ulcers. Low hydrochloric acid (HCl), low immunity and a poor acidic diet can make you more prone to picking it up. It can be associated with childhood asthma and can lead to inflammatory bowel disease. Eating more alkaline foods, mentioned later, and including more thyme and cinnamon as well as meadowsweet and liquorice teas in the diet can help. Cooking with thyme, cinnamon, turmeric and taking grapefruit seed extract can help.

Hypoglycemia is a blood sugar problem that often arises from the dietary extremes that can also lead to diabetes. Insulin production needs to be controlled by avoiding sugars and eating complex carbohydrates and protein. Eating healthy food every 3 hours helps. It often causes severe mood changes, poor concentration and shakiness.

Irritable bowel this can include a range of symptoms including cramping, bloating and constipation alternating with diarrhoea and gas. This can be caused by stress, food intolerances, a poor diet and lack of certain nutrients like magnesium. I find this is often misdiagnosed and all too often there is something else going on that causes these symptoms, like parasites or inflammation. Aloe vera and slippery elm can be useful aids as well as magnesium rich foods and fermented foods.

Liver is implicated in several bowel complaints. A healthy amount of bile is necessary for the intestines. Pale stools can indicate a lack of bile; sometimes constipation is caused by the liver. Dandelion root tea (1-2 cups a day) helps bile flow.

Parasites, constipation, allergies and candida - due to their complexity are talked about in more detail in Ch.5.

Reflux is stomach acid coming up into the mouth and is made worse by obesity, coffee, alcohol, orange, tomato, smoking, rich food, excessive fat, large meals and chocolate. Meadowsweet tea is helpful.

Small intestine bacterial overgrowth (SIBO) causes chronic bloating and gas and is diagnosed by doing a hydrogen breath test. It is often misdiagnosed and is on the increase. It responds well to the specific carbohydrate diet, gut and psychology diet and elemental diet. Prebiotics are contraindicated. Pancreatic enzymes are often needed. Cinnamon, oregano, garlic and peppermint are helpful. Turmeric helps inflammation and papaya and pineapple help digestion. Cabbage juice helps heal the bowel wall. Probiotic foods are useful, see Ch.9. It is essential to remove all sugars and grains.

Ulcers are usually in the duodenum and cause pain and bloating 3 hours after a meal. Ulcers can be caused by acidity so it is important to consume alkalising foods. Cabbage juice is effective for ulcers. Manuka honey and slippery elm are also effective. Avoid heavy protein, dairy, sugar, alcohol and coffee. Include vegetables, salads and vegetable juices.

Often bowel problems require a doctor's examination. I remember a funny experience in my nursing days, when a group of student doctors were huddled around a professor who was very proud, a bit of a toffee nose and loved his colourful ties. As he was showing them how to do a rectal examination the top of his tie went in with his finger. To save embarrassment and the patient knowing, one of the sensitive and bold students quietly cut his tie!

Antibiotics are greatly overused and have caused havoc in the gut of many people. Many years ago I was put on antibiotics for acne which had a very damaging effect on my gut. Skin problems often clear up once the digestive system is working effectively and the diet is healthy. Once you have antibiotics you need to take flora forever, or have fermented foods mentioned later in this book. Fermented foods are a powerful way to start balancing your gut ecology and they are explained in Ch.9.

Antibiotics kill off the good bugs as well as the bad bugs. Without the good bugs you are more susceptible to pathogens and candida. You also start to crave foods that feed candida like yeast and sugar. The lack of good bugs causes gas, fermentation and putrefaction and is known as Dysbiosis. This benefits greatly from a detox mentioned later in the book.

Lack of good bugs makes you susceptible to bugs like clostridium and staphylococci which can lead to colitis.

Other gastrointestinal conditions will all benefit from the advice in this book.

Leaky Gut

This is a very common condition that people often don't know they have. Over a period of time due to damage, the gut lining can become disrupted from constant irritation allowing food molecules to pass through the tiny holes in the bowel lining and leak into the blood stream. A healthy mucosal lining in the gut provides a barrier and houses an extensive number of immune cells. This increased permeability of the gut or intestine allows bacteria, toxins and food to leak into the bloodstream via the cells of the gut lining. The intestinal lining can then be damaged by the passage of these substances, which can cause it to become inflamed and damaged. These inflammatory cells can travel anywhere in the body where there is connective tissue, for example the brain, the lungs and muscles. Lack of minerals gives rise to more inflammation and bad bacteria in the bowel feeds the inflammation. This alarms the immune system and something called immunoglobulins are produced. These immunoglobulins are known as antibodies which are set up to attack these particles called antigens as though they were a poison. This can mean that every time you eat the suspected food your immune system puts alarm bells on as it recognises these particles as foreign and produces antibodies to attack the food (antigen). Then, when you eat that food again the antibodies keep attacking as they have seen that food particle as harmful (a known criminal by the body) and this sets off allergic reactions.

Leaky gut is common after intestinal infections, non-steroidal anti-inflammatory drugs, coeliac and crohn's disease. It is also common in people with AIDS. In crohn's there is a relation to the severity of the disease and the degree of permeability.

Allergies can also occur as this reaction to the particles leaking into the blood stream takes place. Leaking toxins can also damage the liver, which can become overworked and valuable nutrients and other blood components may be also be lost, which over time will result in you becoming run down and lethargic.

A simple whole food diet is necessary to allow the gut lining to heal. Foods containing zinc like sunflower and pumpkin seeds, plain yoghurt, kefir and aloe vera all help. A detox is beneficial as discussed later in the book; the foods in the kitchen pharmacy, recipes and fermented food chapters will all help.

You can have a test done by your naturopath to determine if you have a leaky gut and usually herbs and nutrients are used as part of the healing process but diet is a key factor for healing. Taking all processed foods, gluten and sugars out of the diet helps it to heal as well as having foods high in antioxidants and introducing ferments (see Ch.9).

There are a variety of potential symptoms of leaky gut syndrome, which can include: abdominal pain, eczema, insomnia, fatigue, bloating, stress, anxiety, irritability, food intolerances, malnutrition and muscle cramps. It has also been linked to patients who suffer from crohn's disease and coeliac disease.

The following diagram explains leaky gut. When food particles pass through a leaky gut they are abnormally large; normally they wouldn't get through a gut that wasn't leaky.

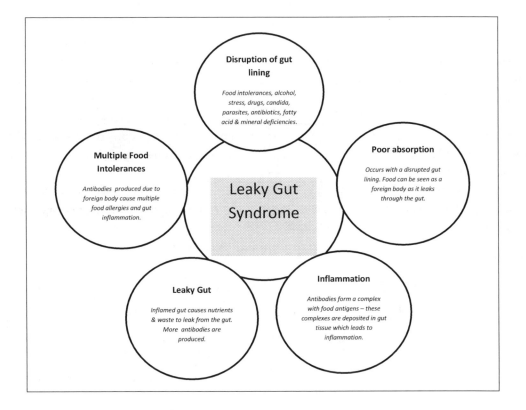

Insulin resistance is a condition where cells in the body fail to respond to the normal actions of the hormone, insulin, produced by your pancreas. Insulin's job is to deliver sugar to cells to provide them with energy. When there is insulin resistance your cells are not able to take in glucose, amino acids (from protein) and fatty acids. What happens is glucose, fatty acids and amino acids 'leak' out of the cells. This lowers energy production. Your body produces more insulin to try to deal with it; too much insulin in the blood stops you using up stored fat and makes you more prone to obesity.

Certain cell types such as fat and muscle cells require insulin to absorb glucose. When these cells fail to respond adequately to circulating insulin, blood glucose levels rise.

Your liver helps regulate glucose levels by reducing its secretion of glucose in the presence of insulin. This normal reduction in the liver's glucose production may not occur in people with insulin resistance.

When your pancreas has to keep putting out insulin it gets exhausted and you are on the path to type 2 Diabetes. Poor carbohydrates such as white flour, white rice, potato, excess milk and sugar can contribute to insulin resistance. An excess of carbohydrates turns to sugar which turns into fat. More insulin is produced and this is also toxic to the brain. Lack of exercise, excessive worry and obesity contribute to insulin resistance. You can become obese due to insulin resistance and conversely you can also become insulin resistant if you are obese. Polycystic ovarian syndrome (PCOS) is caused by insulin resistance and this insulin resistance if not managed can lead to cardiovascular problems and diabetes.

A diet low in sugar and carbohydrates but high in green vegetables, protein, cinnamon, fibre, protein, healthy fat and bitter melon helps manage it. Exercise is important to help manage it and a lack of exercise can cause it.

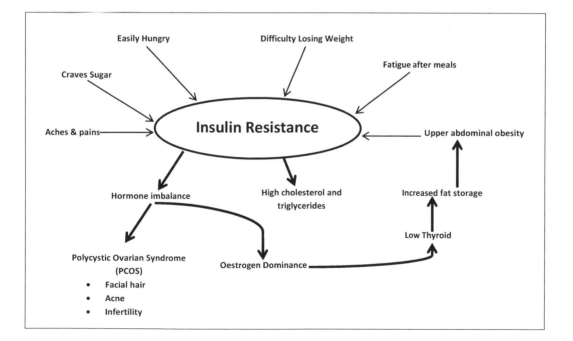

CHAPTER 2

Processing and its effect on the gut

"One should eat to live,
not live to eat."

Anon

CHAPTER 2
Processing and its effect on the gut

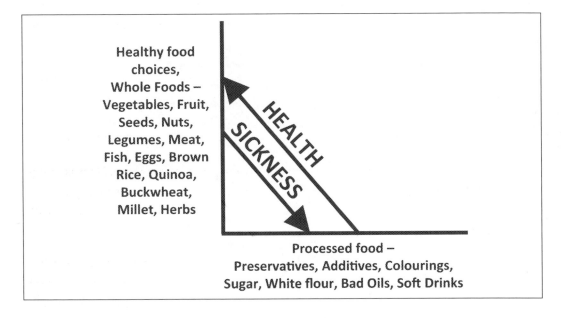

More than 14,000 synthetic chemicals are legally allowed in food production and manufacturing. We were meant to eat whole natural food grown from the earth. Processing has caused so many health problems. Stop paying a fortune to eat things that aren't real food and that will cost you your health and the earth. If you want a guilty pleasure, aim to do it with real food with no hidden nasties. Marketing has fooled you into thinking you can eat guilt free; like putting aspartame into coke, drinking decaf coffee and eating things that look just like butter even though they are definitely not!

We've got more food with all kinds of health claims than ever before and it's not working. We are sicker and fatter than ever. It's got to this because we avoid responsibility, with excuses like "the government wouldn't allow it if it wasn't healthy." Don't wait for everything to be researched hundreds of times and then banned, use your common sense and eat what nature provided. You've slowly been conditioned to believe you can gorge on whatever you want at no cost. You can't, it catches up with even the healthiest of constitutions. Avoid low carb, no fat, lite and de-this and that; it's a con. You've become too invested in other things in life and turned away from the priority of good nourishment. Why buy an expensive plasma T.V. and not invest in high quality food? People complain organic is too expensive, yet they have no problems paying 200 odd dollars for curls, waves and highlights in their hair. Really, do you have to upgrade your car and eat trash? Your body will thank you for reprioritising your values.

What can you do without health? Lie in front of your plasma T.V. all day? You can gorge all you like on bright red lollies, blue drinks, artificially flavoured chips, a melted cheese like substance, white bread that is high in fibre and low-carb beer but eventually you'll feel the pain of it and finally reach for that bowl of fruit and delicious fresh vegetables and find they aren't so bad after all!

Even when your food isn't processed you are getting 20% fewer nutrients compared to what many of your grandparents got (100 years ago). Fertilisers have leached the soils of minerals and only 3 minerals are put back into it. There are 1 billion organisms in a gram of soil and the plants need these to be able to take up nutrients effectively for them to benefit humans.

Alarmingly, parts of America and Europe are having big problems in graveyards because bodies aren't breaking down and remain preserved from all that rubbish in food that stops natural bacteria breaking down waste. At least 40 of the largest graveyards in Germany including ones in Cologne, Munich and Kiel, are no longer usable as they are full to capacity with bodies that have not decayed. Similar problems are being reported in Austria and Switzerland.

"Bodies that were put into the ground 30 years ago look like they went in last week," said Walter Muller, an undertaker in Berlin. "It's like they've been pickled in preservatives and there is no explanation for it."

Leading scientists have been brought in to determine what is going wrong.

"Graves have always been shared or reused. New bodies are added to the grave and nature has its way," said Professor Rainer Horn, head of the department of soil culture at the Christian-Albrechts University in Kiel.

For centuries, gravediggers have reopened plots to bury new coffins, knowing previous coffins buried there will have collapsed into the soil, along with the bodies they contained.

Previously that process would take from 8 to 10 years now however, in approximately one third of graves in Germany, it is taking longer. The crisis is severe and it's thought that people are consuming so many preservatives that their bodies may not be decaying as before. Another belief is that the earth-born bacteria needed in the decomposition process are being wiped out by pollution or pesticides and the level of heavy metals in the soil, such as amalgam used in dental fillings, has been rising in cemeteries, according to tests. I hope that news makes you want to eat more fresh whole food!

Why did it begin?

Firstly, everything post-harvest is defined as food processing so this includes transport, cleaning, blending, preserving by cooking, packaging, marketing and storage.

Food is processed because it decays due to microbes and processing arrests decay. It has enabled food to be transported all over the world to different geographical areas.

Some methods of preservation are not bad, such as using a fridge to slow down microbial growth. Freezing means food can be stored for a year, with a small loss of nutrients when the food is thawed. Canning some foods like tomatoes enables them to be eaten all year round however, you will find canning changes the texture and quality of the food. Pasteurising (for milk, juice and many cans) by heating at temperatures of 80°C for 5 seconds extends shelf life but destroys nutrients.

When food is subjected to high temperatures there is a decrease in the biological value of protein. Changes to smell, colour, taste and texture also occur. Vegetables will lose 20-50% of carotenes, 80% of vitamin C and 60% of B vitamins.

Breakfast cereals and snack foods are heat treated and lose 90% of B vitamins and other nutrients, so vitamins are added back into the product with the illusion that it's packed with vitamins. Why not cook a nice bowl of natural porridge instead? You can prepare it the night before or cook it in a slow cooker or whilst you are having a shower.

When you eat **white bread**, 80% of the nutrition of wholemeal bread is lost. White bread then becomes an anti-nutrient as it uses up more nutrition to digest it than it contains. It is highly acidic which is a precursor to disease and it commonly causes constipation.

Hydrogenated oils also known as trans fats are bad news. Margarine was thought to be healthy by lowering fat however it is now widely recognised (see Ch.8) as harmful to the body and some studies show it is carcinogenic.

Vegetables are best bought fresh rather than frozen or in tins and if you place them in an airtight bag or container before storing them in the fridge they will last a lot longer. Alarmingly, 20% of Americans (which is 1 in 5) eat no fruits or vegetables in their diet and less than 30% have 5 pieces of fruit and vegetables a day!

There are positive methods of processing that enhance nutrients like fermentation (tempeh), pickling or marinating discussed in Chapter 9.

So, the message is to keep away from everything artificial, your body was not designed for it. Many artificial substances have been called safe only to find years later that extensive studies (e.g. pesticides) prove how harmful they are. Don't wait for the studies, just eat what comes from nature.

Food additives - a curse

This is where modern health problems can occur however, in years gone by additives helped preserve food by using natural substances like salt, honey, herbs, spices, chalk and vinegar.

Now additives are used to bulk up foods and add flavour and colour to poor quality foods. In Australia the ANZFA determines what is safe and what is not and additives are classified and coded. Food additives, colours and preservatives are there to make your food last longer, taste better and look better but they can cause hardship for your gut and the rest of your health.

There are over 364 additives (in Australia) including acidity regulators, anti-caking agents, antioxidants, sweeteners, bleaching agents, bulking agents, colouring, flavours, stabilisers, propellants, thickeners, enzymes, minerals, vitamins and preservatives.

So what are they all about?

Food additives are listed according to their functional or class names. It is hard to distinguish the difference between a natural preservative like vitamin C and an artificial one as they are all coded on food packaging by E numbers. However there are only a few natural additives.

Anti-foaming agents

Substances that stop foaming and frothing E 990-999 e.g. in vegetable oils such as dimethylpolysiloxane E 900

Anti-caking agents

Substances that prevent food clumping together like flour and salt E 500-599 such as silicon dioxide E 551

Acidity regulators

Substances that lower the pH of the food and lower the risk of microbial growth E 310-399 such as metatartic acid E 353

Antioxidants that are natural are vitamin C, E 300 and vitamin E, E 306

Bleaching agents These are used to whiten flour E 920-929 e.g. E 926

Bulking agents These add bulk to food e.g. E 1400

Emulsifiers They help form emulsion e.g. E 440-449 are natural emulsifiers

Flour agents help the shelf life of flours and are commonly used in breads E 510-519 e.g. aluminium chloride E 510

Food acids help control browning and add gel and tartness to jams

Glazing agents can be natural, like beeswax. They add a polish to the outside of fruit

Preservatives help stop unfriendly bacteria destroying food E 200-299 e.g. benzoic acid E 221

Propellants are gases put into containers to allow a whipped effect with creams and toppings

Raising agents add gas to bottles and raise breads

Artificial sweeteners - sweet poisons (see Ch. 11 Kitchen Pharmacy for healthy sweet alternatives)

They have been shown to cause behavioural problems and can be carcinogenic. There are several sweeteners used regularly which include:

Saccharin

It is used in diet products, soft drinks and chewing gum.

- It has been shown to cause: Uterine, ovarian, skin, blood vessel and other organ cancer in rodents.

- It increases the potency of other cancer causing chemicals.

- It can cause bladder cancer. The best epidemiology study (National Cancer Institute) found that the use of artificial sweeteners (saccharin and cyclamate) were associated with a higher incidence of bladder cancer.

Aspartame

It is used in diet foods, soft drinks, drink mixes, gelatine desserts, frozen desserts and packet food.

- There is debate over its potential behavioural effects and effects on cancer.

- It can cause dizziness, headaches and hallucinations.

- There is a rare metabolic disease called PKU- phenyleketonuria. People who have this need to avoid it.

Sucralose

This is another artificial sweetener. Most sucralose that is eaten is not broken down by the body, so it has no calories. It is also known by the E number 955. Sucralose is about 600 times as sweet as sucrose (table sugar), twice as sweet as saccharin and three times as sweet as aspartame. It can be used in baking or in products that require a longer shelf life. The success of sucralose-based products is its favourable comparison to other low-calorie sweeteners in terms of taste, stability and safety. Common brand names of sucralose-based sweeteners are Splenda, Sukrana, SucraPlus. It is found in a huge number (4500) of foods and drinks. Sucralose has not been shown to be carcinogenic however, it is artificial and it has been shown to reduce healthy flora in the gut by up to 50%. In animals it has been shown to shrink the thymus gland and it has been shown to cause migraines in some people.

Fructose although natural it is important to avoid this for many gut problems (see Ch.6)

Sugar more addictive than cocaine!

Sugar although natural, is highly processed and is the most destructive substance you can eat. It is the biggest single dietary killer as it sucks minerals out of the body, plays havoc with insulin and causes obesity. Back in 2007 a revealing study titled "Intense sweetness surpasses cocaine reward" found that when rats were given the option of choosing between water sweetened with saccharin or cocaine, the large majority (94%) preferred the sweet taste of saccharin. The same preference was found with sucrose. The preference for saccharin was not overcome by increasing doses of cocaine. In other studies, bees and insects respond in a similar way.

Sugar is also more addictive than cigarettes and alcohol but the less you have the less you want. Sugar is added to so many foods for taste and as a preservative as it increases the osmotic gradient in food. This dries out the food and without water, microbes cannot survive.

Reduce your sugar

There is a high risk of diabetes, developing bad bacteria in your gut and you have a 50% higher chance of heart attack and stroke if you have high blood sugar levels. You are more at risk if you don't exercise. In 1900 the average person ate 5kg of sugar per year now it's increased to 75kg and it's extremely destructive to health.

So what else does sugar do?

It increases free radicals, reduces vitamin C uptake, lowers immunity, decreases an important nutrient called nitric oxide in the arteries and stops clots from breaking down. It destroys healthy flora in your gut and makes you more open to contracting candida and parasites. Sugar feeds these nasties. It also affects the collagen in your artery walls, which makes them more rigid and less able to expand and contract; this then easily attracts plaque which blocks the arteries.

10 ways to reduce sugar

1. Eat more protein, fibre and good fat like coconut, avocado and almonds.

2. Take out white sugar, white flour and white rice. Reduce your carbohydrates generally.

3. Eat foods high in chromium which helps improve insulin efficiency e.g. eggs.

4. Increase foods high in vitamin C like berries, lemons, limes, parsley and red capsicum.

5. Eat more magnesium rich foods like buckwheat and brown rice, especially if sugar cravings occur before periods.

6. De-stress without using food. Call a friend, have an aromatherapy bath, go for a walk, indulge in a hobby or a good book.

7. Ginseng tea, mulberry leaf tea and bitter melon in cooking help lower blood sugar.

8. The herb saffron also helps curb sugar cravings

9. Exercise using a combination of cardiovascular, resistance and stretching exercises.

10. Get everything out of the house that contains sugar. Don't worry about the kids, your husband or your wife; it's not good for them either! Put it all in the bin.

Colouring

There are natural colours and synthetic colours that are put into food (E 100-199). The natural colours are from fruits or vegetables and include anthocyanins, porphyrins (which are blue and purple) and carotenoids which are orange. Turmeric and beetroot can be used as natural colourings.

Some synthetic colours are potentially carcinogenic and are associated with behavioural problems in children. Reactions to these colours are not always apparent until a large portion of the population has had them. Sunset yellow has been banned in the U.S. because of associated health problems.

Many people have allergic reactions to synthetic colours and more so if they are allergic to salicylates. The reactions can range from asthma to rashes and nasal inflammation. Synthetic coal tar dyes put a demand on the liver when they are metabolised and are best avoided.

Flavours

They modify the flavours in food (E 600-699). Some flavours are natural but a lot aren't like monosodium glutamate (MSG) E 621, which is a common flavouring used in restaurants (especially in Chinese food) and it's common in snack food. On packets it can be called flavour enhancer or natural flavour enhancer which is misleading. Common reactions are headaches, dizziness, breathing difficulties and tightness in the jaw and back.

Sodium nitrite is a preservative colouring and flavouring which stabilises the red colour in cured meats. It is in bacon, ham, hot dogs, smoked fish and corned beef. It can lead to cancer causing chemicals known as nitrosamines. The use of sodium nitrite has lessened as refrigeration has been shown to preserve these meats. Some companies have added vitamin C to bacon to stop nitrosamines from forming. Nitrites also occur when you burn your toast and on chargrilled or barbequed meat, so throw it out if it burns. Sodium nitrate is not to be confused with nitrite, though the name is similar, as it is an antimicrobial preservative.

Food additive reactions

One study of food additives on Attention Deficit Disorder (ADD) found that artificial colouring or sodium benzoate or both in the diet, increased hyperactivity in children. There is a lot of evidence that shows food additives cause behavioural changes as well as gut problems and eczema. Having a nutrient dense diet with lots of fruit and vegetables and good amounts of water, stops reactions. The health of the intestines and liver also plays a big part in stopping or preventing reactions.

Adverse reactions of hyperactive children to various foods and chemicals

Studies have shown that many hyperactive children react to foods as well as additives. These children usually have gut problems that are not diagnosed. The additives foods that cause the highest number of reactions are colourings and preservatives, soy, cow's milk, chocolate, grapes, wheat, oranges, cow's cheese, eggs and peanuts. Naturopathic work on the gut can often resolve these problems as well as having a healthy diet and lifestyle.

Food Standard Australia New Zealand carries out safety assessments of food additives before they are allowed to be used. The following things are checked:

Is the food additive safe (at the required level in that particular food)?

Are there good technological reasons for the use of the food additive?

Will consumers be clearly informed about its presence?

Unfortunately some reactions are not known until a large portion of the population has been eating them.

If you eat whole foods you don't need to worry about additives and better still, organic food has no harmful additives besides, foods that have additives are generally dead with no life force nor do they have any great nutrient value. Refined food like white flour, processed food, fast food, stale food and stimulants like sugar are depleted in nutrition and life force. It is best to avoid these foods and eat more fruit, vegetables, sprouted grains, seeds, kefir, plain yoghurt and fresh vegetable juices. It's not so hard to eat a piece of fruit or a few sunflower seeds or some plain yoghurt. If you cook at low temperatures not only does the food taste nicer it is more nutrient dense. Having a slow cooker makes this easy. A great way to cook meat is to put it on a really low temperature C 80-100 all night or day. I've done this recently and the meat is amazingly tender and tasty.

Milk

So many people today are lacking in calcium and it's probable that you are too. We have an extraordinary amount of unnecessary osteoporosis in the western world and yet we eat so much calcium (this is partly due to an acidic diet). The way modern milk is processed with pasteurisation is an assault on the body as calcium is poorly absorbed.

A study was done in Australia where 100 calves were fed their mother's milk and another 100 calves fed pasteurised milk. The calves were killed at 6 months and all 100 of the calves fed pasteurised milk had osteoporosis. When pasteurisation happens it destroys phosphatase which is an enzyme that governs the uptake of calcium. Vitamin D is also needed to set up the receptors in the gut to absorb calcium. You can buy unpasteurised milk from some organic shops or you can get shares in a local cow and collect your own unpasteurised milk! See chapter 11 for calcium rich bone broth.

So what are a lot of people lacking due to processed foods?

Protein and lack of it causes fatigue and it's important for neurotransmitter production in the brain and enzyme production for the digestion.

Iron in meat, beetroot and greens is important for red blood cell production and its absorption is disrupted by tea, coffee, alcohol and other substances. It also requires vitamin C for absorption.

Vitamin C in fruits and some vegetables is a common deficiency and you can easily be tested in naturopathic clinics. It is water soluble so lost from the body every day. It is really important for adrenal health and as mentioned for iron absorption.

B Vitamins in whole grains are lacking in many people because of processed and overcooked foods and excessive stress. B vitamins have multiple functions in energy pathways and mood regulation.

Antioxidants in fruits and vegetables are often missing because of food processing and also excess toxins in your body. Vitamins A, C, E and selenium are lost in processing.

As you can see many nutrients may be deficient if the diet is high in packaged, processed, overcooked and reheated foods and there is an absence of whole, fresh living food.

Beware of diet food that says fat free or virtually fat free. Many products that are labelled fat free never had any fat in them, like soups. A lot of reduced fat biscuits are high in sugar. Products marked light/lite usually refer to the colour like olive oil or to the salt content. You generally put on weight because of high carbohydrates or sugar and if you don't have enough good fat you will crave these fat making foods. Think about how goats cheese, avocado, coconut oil, nuts and seeds help you feel full and this stops you eating sugars and excess carbohydrates.

Improve dietary choices

So how do you improve your choices?

There are several things you can do like going to health events, healthy cooking classes and getting advice from natural health practitioners. One of the most important things is planning and organising your food ahead of time. Pick one day to work out what you will need for the week to make healthy choices. If you have foods like a hummus dip, carrots, celery, avocado, fruit and nuts in the fridge then you are less likely to go for biscuits or chocolate because you have nothing in the fridge. Better still, have no bad food in the house. Allow yourself time to shop, select healthy food, prepare and eat your food. To be honest I don't bother with anything that has additives; it's easier to get whole natural food than be constantly scanning E numbers on packets and tins. This is a good website if you do need to know how to read a label: www.wikihow.com/Read-Nutrition-Facts-on-Food-Labels.

There are several organic companies that home deliver such as Victoria organic delivery and natural healthy home delivery takeaways.

When you shop, utilise quality ingredients, emphasising fresh natural foods. It's amazing what bad habits you may have got into with processed and packaged foods.

As a teenager, I lived a short time with an Indonesian family in Bali. On my birthday they made me a savoury cake. It was a mound of yellow rice dyed with turmeric and it had thin strips of omelette all around it and coloured vegetables. Sweet things weren't a part of their diet and every food was whole and unprocessed. The teenagers couldn't afford alcohol and spent their evenings playing drafts, chess, singing and playing musical instruments.

Oh it was so different from western life with teenagers eating junk food, consuming lots of soft drink, alcohol and cigarettes. We have a lot to learn to get back to the basics of healthy living.

To get in touch with food start to grow it, even if you grow it in your kitchen like sprouts and wheat grass. Food can be grown in pots on balconies. You can also make your own yoghurt, kefir and cultured vegetables. This will get you in touch with nature and inspire you to eat more natural clean foods.

For most people include some raw food, to help more live enzymes stimulate your digestion and cook at low temperatures to help the life force of food. Most of all, enjoy your food. Enjoy the tastes, colours, flavours and aromas you create. The secret of a good salad is to always have a fresh herb and tasty healthy dressing. For example mint, basil or coriander added and a dressing of olive oil, lemon juice and garlic or tamari, lifts the flavour and adds zest.

When you eat whole food, your digestion will love it. Your body will feel more alive and everything will work better. Get rid of refined, processed, convenience foods and stimulants as they all deplete your life force. Get rid of white food as it takes more nutrition to digest it than it contains. That is why we call this and sugar anti-nutrients.

Avoid being sucked in by food advertising as it's all about processed foods and uses imagery to manipulate you into believing it's good for you.

Constant unresolved stress will have an impact on your digestion and nervous system and disturb many metabolic processes. If you eat well you will cope better with stress and if you manage stress your digestion will be more efficient. If you are stressed, avoid eating until you feel calmer, as you just won't digest your food efficiently. Think about doing something for relaxation like yoga, meditation and tai chi.

If you start to fill your pantry and fridge with whole fresh foods and take out processed foods and if you prepare and cook in a wholesome way, your digestion will love it and thank you for it.

CHAPTER 3

The benefits of organic food and the dangers of pesticides and genetic engineering

*"Health is not valued
till sickness comes."*

Dr. Thomas Fuller
(1654-1734)

CHAPTER 3
The benefits of organic food and the dangers of pesticides and genetic engineering

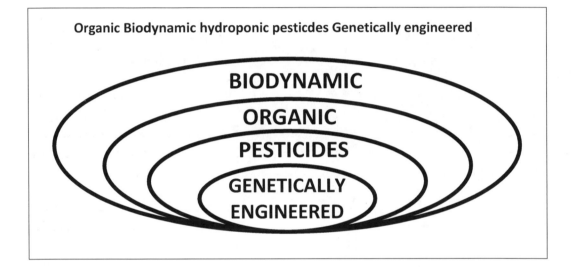

Organic Biodynamic hydroponic pesticdes Genetically engineered

BIODYNAMIC

ORGANIC

PESTICIDES

GENETICALLY ENGINEERED

Organic food

Does organic food really make a difference? Yes, but at first it's not obvious. Accumulating toxins from pesticides and herbicides has a big impact on your digestion and the rest of your body over time. The liver continually detoxes chemicals from food and the environment on a day to day basis however, there is only so much it can take.

There are many studies that show large amounts of pesticides in the umbilical cords of newborn babies and in the fat cells of adults. Another reason to buy organic is that a lot of foods are irradiated and people think it's better than pesticide use but irradiation has its own health problems. Organic food could extend your life and research has shown this to be true in animals.

Irradiated food is when the food is treated with ionising radiation to halt the spoilage of food and destroy micro-organisms. Even though the food does not become radioactive there is concern amongst the public and consumer advocacy groups like Public Citizen that vitamins are lost, good micro-organisms may be lost and chemical changes to the food may occur that are harmful to the consumer. Irradiation is used in 50 countries on 500,000 metric tons of food worldwide.

Isn't it best to invest in your health now to save ill health and cost in the future?

Think about your children

I know one family who sacrificed buying a home to feed their children with the best organic food. Those children are adults today and have no health problems and an abundance of energy. Now I'm not saying you have to go that far, many people won't have to sacrifice their house but just look at other ways you can budget to get good healthy food. Join local food co-ops. Steiner schools often have cheaper organic food markets. Markets often have organic food at great value. Farmers markets often sell great value, pesticide free food that hasn't yet been labelled organic.

One mother said to me when she started buying organic food, her son came home and only ate one apple instead of three. He was getting more nutrients in the one organic apple, minus the chemicals.

A study of 8 different non organic baby foods produced by Gerber, Heinz and Beech-Nut showed residues of 16 different pesticides including brain toxins and hormone disrupters. With a good blender it's easy to make your own baby food. You can freeze it in ice cube trays for smaller portions.

In another study at the University of Washington, pesticide breakdown products were analysed in pre-school aged children and the researchers found that children eating organic fruits and vegetables had six times fewer pesticide remnants than children eating conventional produce. The study compared concentrations of organophosphorus (OP) pesticides (they disrupt the nervous system) in the urine of 39 children aged 2-4 years old. The findings showed parents could easily reduce their children's chemical load by giving them organic food. Children are more at risk from pesticide contamination because they eat more relative to their body mass and they eat foods higher in pesticides which include juices, fruits and vegetables. Another study of 96 children showed OP pesticides in all but one child who was on an exclusively organic diet. It's worth thinking about investing in their long term health and saving money on medical bills down the track. You will also add to your child's vitality, learning ability and emotional state by feeding them organic food.

You can save money

Others have said they save on packaged food when going organic. The food industry makes most of its money on food products rather than original produce like grains, nuts, seeds, vegetables and fruits. So it is much cheaper, for example, to make porridge from raw organic oats than to buy a packet of commercial cereal that has been processed and is often full of sugar. You will also find the porridge keeps you full for longer. Now you may think, oh but the porridge takes so long to make. Soak it overnight in water or whatever organic milk you like. It could be rice milk, oat milk, almond milk, goat's milk or cow's milk. Then you'll find it's a lot quicker to cook and you can do it whilst you are in the shower.

If you have a slow cooker, you can cook it overnight. See the recipes at the back for breakfast ideas. A slow cooker is a wonderful investment and I used to use it a lot when I was a student. If you are busy in the morning you can chop a few vegetables, throw in a pulse or brown rice and a few herbs, or make a soup and when you come home in the evening it's all cooked and the house smells of delicious home cooking.

Other benefits of buying organic

Buying organic helps the environment, increases your nutrition and the taste is better. You also don't have the burden of toxic chemicals.

The biggest study into organic food found that it is more nutritious than ordinary produce and may help to lengthen the quality of people's lives.

The evidence from the £12 million, four-year project will end years of debate and is likely to overturn government advice that eating organic food is no more than a lifestyle choice.

The study found that organic fruit and vegetables contained as much as 40% more antioxidants, which scientists believe can cut the risk of cancer and heart disease, Australia's biggest killers. They also had higher levels of beneficial minerals such as iron and zinc.

Professor Carlo Leifert, the co-ordinator of the European Union-funded project, said the differences were so marked that organic produce would help to increase the nutrient intake of people not eating the recommended five portions a day of fruit and vegetables. "If you have just 20% more antioxidants and you can't get your kids to do five a day, then you might be o.k. with four a day," he said.

Leifert said, "There is enough evidence now that the level of good things is higher in organics."

A group of researchers grew fruit and vegetables and reared cattle on adjacent organic and nonorganic sites on a 725 acre farm attached to Newcastle University, England, and at other sites in Europe. They found that levels of antioxidants in milk from organic herds were up to 90% higher than in milk from conventional herds.

As well as finding up to 40% more antioxidants in organic vegetables, they also found that organic tomatoes from Greece had significantly higher levels of antioxidants, including flavonoids thought to reduce coronary artery disease.

Grow your own

For those of you interested in growing your own food www.plantagenda.com.au is very good for companion planting, so that you can grow foods that help each other and minimise pests. It also tells you what vegetables to plant in what months.

Companion planting that I have found useful incudes growing chamomile around plants to act as a natural fungicide and it helps prevent pests.

In general, herbs grown around vegetables prevent pests.

Tomatoes do well when planted with basil and parsley and asparagus. They don't work well with potato (as it's the same family) or with rosemary.

Borage easily increases resistance to tomatoes, strawberries and seeds.

You can also use a disco ball instead of a scarecrow; it's just as good for scaring the birds. For organic seeds and lots of garden tips I'd highly recommend www.diggers.com.au and www. edenseeds.com.au

When you go to buy organic food you want to make sure it's certified.

There are three organisations in Australia:

Association for Sustainable Agriculture Australia under the N.A.S.A.A. label.

Biological Farmers of Australia under the B.F.A. label.

Bio-Dynamic Farmers of Australia under the Demeter label.

The three levels are:

"Organic," being complete organic production with no artificial fertilisers or synthetic chemicals for more than two years. This is preferable.

"Conversion," being complete organic production for less than 2 years.

"Sustainable," being almost complete organic production with a minimum of low toxicity sprays that have been used under strict guidelines.

Organic farmers rely on:

- Sound rotations

- Natural nitrogen fixation

- Biologically active soil life

- Recycled farm manures and crop residues

- Appropriate cultivation

- Biological pest control

- Ethical livestock systems

Organic farmers do not use:

- Synthetic fertilisers

- Synthetic pesticides or herbicides

- Growth regulators or promoters

- Antibiotic and hormonal stimulants

- Intensive livestock systems

Why farm organically?

Organic farming produces food that has optimal quality using methods which seek to co-exist with and not dominate natural systems.

There is clear evidence that conventional agriculture has led to:

- Damage to the environment

- Loss of wild life diversity

- Loss of wild life habitat such as hedge rows

- Potentially hazardous residue in our food

- Ethically unacceptable livestock systems

- Damage to soil structure and fertility

- Increasing economic burden to society

- Overuse of non-renewable resources

- Organic farming helps to avoid these problems

Some good reasons to buy organic

It's really worth embarking on having organic food for a minimum of 3 months and observing the difference in your well-being as well as the taste and texture of the food.

- Improved taste - it is less watery with more intense natural sweetness.

- Improved nutrient status. Organic farmers add fewer nitrates (carcinogens).

- Increased vitamin content. Kelp meal and compost is used which has a high mineral content that goes into the food soil making it a higher quality food than conventional farming.

- Avoidance of artificial chemicals, pesticides and fertilisers. Farm workers handling chemicals exhibit increased incidence of cancer (stomach, prostate, brain and skin). Pesticides can mimic hormones interrupting normal function of the endocrine (hormonal) system, contributing to the rise of breast cancer in females, ovarian cancer and prostate cancer in males. Those nasty chemicals are also a lot of work for your digestive system to keep trying to detoxify.

- Absence of genetically modified organisms.

- Emphasis on animal welfare. Cruel practices avoided.

- Animals grown without the use of antibiotics and hormones.

- Methods of production are based on sustainability, wildlife and the environment.

- Reduces risk of mad cow disease in humans consuming organic beef.

- Utilises modern science and ecology whilst using traditional farming methods.

- By supporting these farmers it will encourage growth and the price will then go down.

Organic crop rotation

A sound rotation is an essential component of the organic farm. It balances fertility, building and cropping and provides the principle means of weed, pest and disease control.

A good organic crop rotation involves:

- A balance between nitrogen fixing crops and nitrogen demanding crops.

- Alternating between deep and shallow rooting crops.

- Covering crops to keep the soil protected where possible.

- Balancing crops which supress and are susceptible to weeds and balancing crops with different pest and disease susceptibility.

- Balance of seasonal labour requirements and availability.

Biodynamic farming

This type of farming is even better than organic farming. Organic farming helps stop the devastation caused by humans but it doesn't give back to the earth in the same way as biodynamic farming does.

Biodynamics is part of the work of Rudolf Steiner known as anthroposophy - a new approach to science which integrates observation of natural phenomena and knowledge of the spirit. It treats the earth as a living being taking into account the forces of nature and picking and planting at specific times. It takes into account the cosmic rhythms of the sun, moon and planets and how that affects sowing, cultivating and harvesting.

One of biodynamics fundamental efforts is to build up stable humus in our soil through composting. We gain our health and strength from the breaking down of the food we eat and how we assimilate it. The more vital our food, the more it helps our own energy. Biodynamic farmers and gardeners therefore, aim for quality.

Chemical farming has developed short-cuts to quantity by adding soluble minerals to the soil. The plants take these up via water, by-passing their normal way of seeking from the soil what is needed for health, growth and vital force. This results in a dead soil and artificially stimulated growth.

Biodynamic farming grows food with a strong connection to a healthy, living soil and biodynamic preparations are used to enhance the nutrient status of the soil.

Plant and animal materials are put together in specific recipes in certain seasons of the year and then placed in compost piles. Two of the preparations are used directly in the field, one on the earth before planting, to stimulate soil life and one on the leaves of plants to improve their capacity to receive the light. These preparations have been scientifically verified to have beneficial effects on the plants and soil.

A farm works with the preservation and recycling of the life-forces. Vegetable waste, manure, leaves and food scraps all contain valuable vitality which can be held and used for building up the soil if they are handled well, so composting is a key activity in biodynamic work.

Steiner stressed the absurdity of agricultural economics determined by people who have never raised crops or managed a farm.

Pesticides

Synthetic pesticides have been used since the 1930s. Organochlorine pesticides were used starting in the 1940s. Some uses include agriculture and forestry as well as protecting wooden buildings. In the 1970s, another group of insecticides was introduced. A pesticide is any substance or mixture of substances used to destroy, suppress or alter the life cycle of any pest.

Pesticides have been found in the fat tissue and blood of humans and more research is showing the harm that they do. Endosulfan is an insecticide that is gradually being banned globally because of its harm to human health. It was banned in Australia in 2012 and amongst other health concerns it was found to affect the human foetus.

Carbendazim is in a range of fruits and macadamia plantations in Australia and has caused infertility and eyesight problems. We are now finding toxic waterways with run off from pesticides;

like people getting sick from water ways and pets dying. Central nervous system problems were widely found in Noosa, Australia after endosulfan used on macadamia plantations affected the Noosa River. It also seemed to cause the death of fish and many fish were found with 2 heads.

The investigation team are not convinced that endosulfan was the cause though evidence heavily points towards it and it has been banned in 50 countries. Australia can sometimes be slow to take action in stopping the risks to human and environmental health. The pesticide DDT was banned some time ago but researchers are still finding it in breast milk.

Pesticides are very carcinogenic and not only are they sprayed on food but in sports grounds and parks. The most highly sprayed plants are:

- Tomatoes - which are sprayed over 30 times during their growth.

- Strawberries - which are sprayed over 25 times during their growth.

- Snow peas - which are sprayed over 20 times during their growth.

- Apples -which are sprayed over 14 times during their growth.

Not only this but more toxins are added post-harvest to enhance ripening, then fungicides and waxes are used and the end products aren't as pretty as they look!

We don't have much control over what is done overseas, for example the delicious lychees you may be eating from a tin produced in Thailand are highly overloaded with toxic spray during their growth cycle.

In a recent study in America 1400 children were tested for 13 commonly used pesticides. All 1400 had unacceptable levels of every pesticide tested. Start eating organic now to avoid the build-up of these toxins later and the impact to your health. It's a lot cheaper to eat organic/biodynamic than have large health bills and suffering later.

More research in Belgium has found that women with breast cancer are six times more likely to have pesticides in their blood stream. Another group of researchers in Hawaii followed 8000 people over 34 years and found that pesticide residue on food significantly raised the risk of Parkinson's disease. It's time to stop eating poison and realise that organic farming has given us many great lessons and it needs your support. You can have diets that are simple, fresh and grown organically. More and more people want to know where their food comes from, how it was processed and what has gone into it and I hope you do too.

Many natural substances can be used as pesticides, such as extracts of pyrethrum, garlic, tea-tree oil and eucalyptus oil. When these natural products are used as pesticides they become subject to the same controls as pesticides produced synthetically. Changing farming methods like companion farming, permaculture and organic farming often removes the need for pesticides.

Genetically modified food

Genetically modified food is replacing one harmful way of farming with pesticides to another harmful way of farming.

Genetically modified food is one of the biggest human experiments and it's proving to be dangerous. Another reason to go organic/biodynamic is to avoid the risk of having genetically modified food on your plate. We have been crossing genes for a long time and this is not necessarily harmful, for example crossing different species of apples to create new types of apples. Historically, farmers bred plants and animals for their desired traits to create wide variations in species.

Genetically modified food (G.M.) is different and it's alarming. No G.M. foods can be classed as organic. It is the artificial insertion of genes and chromosomes within the nuclei of cells. G.M. allows this process to speed up by moving desired genes from one plant to another or from an animal to a plant or vice versa (often unrelated species).

It can be done with plants, animals, food and tomatoes are being crossed with fish to prevent frost bite! An unassuming person with an allergy to fish may eat it and they therefore react to the tomato.

In G.M. crops, genes have been transferred from bacteria, a virus, or other plant to make it more resistant to a chemical, weed killer or to produce its own insecticide. One of the major producers of genetically engineered seed is Monsanto. This organisation claims bioengineering will improve agricultural sustainability by:

- Decreasing the need for herbicides, pesticides and insecticides.

- Reducing tillage and therefore reducing soil erosion.

- Increasing moisture retention and reducing fuel costs and emissions.

- They claim overall that it will improve wildlife habitat around the crop.

Dangers of genetically modified food

There are many concerns around G.M. food such as environmental concerns, health concerns and financial control.

Environmental concerns

- Crossing species boundaries. These boundaries have remained intact for millions of years. We don't yet know the full extent of the consequences of gene manipulation and how do we measure the long term effects if G.M. seeds are blowing across the countryside. Cross pollination doesn't protect native species from the foreign G.M. one. There are risks to organic crops. Wind, rain, birds and insects can carry pollen to adjoining fields; this means that once G.M. seeds are released can they never be recaptured.

- Damage to the food matrix. They can affect insects that may be beneficial.

- Crops with built in insecticides could harm beneficial insects as well as the intended target pests e.g. ladybird and lacewing insects which eat the G.M. created crop can be affected by the insecticide toxin.

- Risk of loss of wild species - they are endangered in this environment.

- If any bioengineered plants or animals are bred to be "superior"- that is hardier, stronger and more robust - they may overpower the wild species. There may be a risk to wild fish if G.M. carp, salmon or trout are released (or escape) - they may be bigger and greedier than their wild counterparts! Who will survive?!

- Creation of G.M. "superweeds" and "superpests" - in time, pests and weeds will develop a resistance to the applied or inbred pesticides/herbicides and more and stronger chemicals will be needed. The creation of new bacteria/viruses may occur.

- Creating resistance in plants to viruses has resulted in the viruses mutating to a more virulent form. One G.M. microorganism (Klebsiellaplanticola) has been found to destroy soil nutrients.

- Increased pesticide residue in soil and on crops. Pesticide and herbicide reduction has been short lived. Benefits for consumers have not materialised. Many G.M. farmers have not used fewer products than conventional farmers and have had to resort to pesticides.

Health concerns

- The G.M. technique could alter and disrupt the normal function of the genes in the crops. Changes in biochemistry pathways may mean toxin production. Also, the novel protein made by the gene could cause allergies which can be fatal for some people.

- Most of these proteins have not been consumed by humans before. Long term testing is required to prevent public health disasters. It is very important that food be labelled with G.M. products, so that those who are at risk can make choices.

- A.R.M. genes (antibiotic resistant markers) The European Union is considering banning foods that contain these altogether! They are linked to foreign genes in plants to determine if the gene slice was successful.

- Some researchers suggest the risk of these recombining with disease causing bacteria or microbes in the environment or in the flesh of animals or people who eat G.M. food and the increased risk of antibiotic resistance in the population, which is already a problem due to overuse of the drug.

Economic control

- There is a global food security threat. G.M. food also uses terminator technology which means after a span of life the plant commits suicide and no new seeds develop for the next generation. The terminator seed or sterile seed will create dependence of farmers (who currently save and reuse seed) on biotech conglomerates who no doubt will escalate costs to this group.

- It creates dependency in poor countries.

- The same companies who produce the G.M. seed also produce the pesticides, so there is a potential for exploitation and profit which may result in even more resistant plants being developed, meaning the farmer will need more herbicide to kill weeds!

- There is a concern of ownership and control by the monopoly of the 5 multi nationals: Monsanto, Aventis, Novartis, AstraZeneca and DuPont who produce 80% of the world's G.M. crops.

- They have patented genes, crops and seeds. They can charge farmers royalties if they wish to resow the seed in the future. 1.4 billion people use seed saved from harvesting for replanting in developing countries. This has pushed out small farmers in countries like India, and who are now unemployed.

Gene splicing has given rise to many concerns. The health and environmental consequences are far from known. The potential risks of G.M. food should not be underestimated and legitimate concerns should not be dismissed as trivial.

What can you do?

- Insist on adequate independent safety guards and controls on corporations.

- Involve the public in decisions on the need for regulation.

- Insist on strict legal liability for transgressions or diverse effects of G.M. foods.

- Ensure all products are labelled so you can make a choice between G.M. and non G.M. foods.

- Help ongoing research into implications on environmental and human health.

- Vote with your dollar and buy organic food. You don't want to be eating G.M. food and popping pills for your tummy problems. Treat your body more kindly.

- If you are in Australia you can join www.geneethics.org. This is a great organisation that campaigns against G.M. foods and is very informative about what is really going on.

- Watch the film www.foodmatters.com

- To see the standard visit www.standard.org.au

- I'd recommend this site for a further look into G.M. and how we can produce food in a healthier and more sustaining way. The site contains many interesting interviews and articles about G.M. For information on G.M. overseas go to, www.inmotionmagazine. com.shiva.html an Indian physicist discusses sustainable agriculture.

More Proof

With further studies we are starting to see more proof that G.M. food is harmful, like colon and other tumours developing and shorter lives occurring; seen in the following study.

In September 2012, *Food and Chemical Toxicology*, an international scientific journal, released a study by a team of scientists at France's Caen University led by Professor Gilles-Eric Seralini.

"Seralini's group based their experiment on the same protocol as the Monsanto study but, critically, were testing more parameters more frequently. The rats were studied for much longer—their full two year average life-time instead of just 90 days as in the Monsanto study. The long time-span proved critical. The first tumours only appeared 4 to 7 months into the study. In industry's earlier 90-day study on the same G.M. maize, Monsanto NK603, signs of toxicity were seen but were dismissed as "not biologically meaningful" by industry and EFSA alike. It seems they were indeed very biologically meaningful."

"Their findings were more than alarming. The Seralini study concluded, "In females, all treated groups died 2–3 times more often than controls, and more rapidly. This difference was visible in 3 male groups fed GMOs...Females developed large mammary tumours almost always more often than and before controls; the pituitary was the second most disabled organ; the sex hormonal balance was modified by GMO and roundup treatments. In treated males, liver congestions and necrosis were 2.5–5.5 times higher. This pathology was confirmed by optic and transmission electron microscopy. Marked and severe kidney nephropathies were also generally 1.3–2.3 times greater. Males presented 4 times more large palpable tumours than controls..."

To read more on this see www.organicconsumers.org/articles/article_26833.cfm

Data shows that the average Australian household spends more on junk food than on fruit and vegetables, more on alcohol than fruit and vegetables and more on takeaways than fruit and vegetables. They also spend five times more on recreation than on fruit and vegetables!

Vote with your dollar

I know a lady, Victoria Boutenko, who was the first person to get a McDonald's cafe closed down but not by petitions or violence; she simply went to every venue she could in a little town outside of Oregon in the U.S. and lectured people on how to eat healthy food. The reduction in demand for McDonald's was so great, that it had to close.

Find out where your local markets, farmers markets and health food shops are. Many companies home deliver organic food which is beneficial if you are time poor and tempted by commercial foods and unhealthy take-aways.

Often you can afford organic food just by reprioritising and you may find that you actually spend less because you save all the money you used to spend on junk food and luxury items. Don't you want to know what's in your food and what it's doing to your precious body? Organic/biodynamic food isn't necessarily extravagant, it's how you are supposed to eat.

CHAPTER 4

Are your pots and pans poisoning you?

"As I see it, every day you do one of two things,
build health or produce disease in yourself."

Adelle David
(1904-1974)

Chapter 4
Are your pots and pans poisoning you?

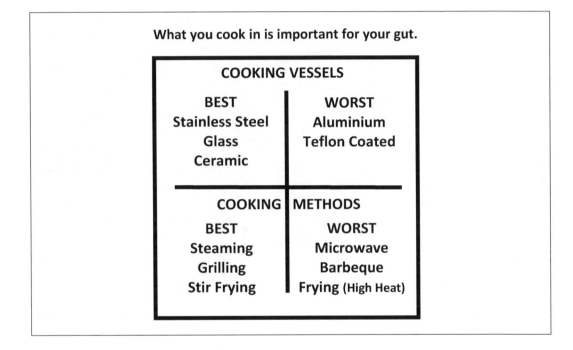

What you cook in is important for your gut.

COOKING VESSELS	
BEST **Stainless Steel** **Glass** **Ceramic**	**WORST** **Aluminium** **Teflon Coated**
COOKING	METHODS
BEST **Steaming** **Grilling** **Stir Frying**	**WORST** **Microwave** **Barbeque** **Frying** (High Heat)

It is important for your digestive system not to have to deal with added toxins. Your body has to deal with enough from daily toxins in the modern world e.g. car fumes, industry fumes, off gassing from carpets, furniture and building materials, toxic foods and drinks.

So have a look around your kitchen at the cookware you have and the plates and utensils you use and ask yourself, is it safe? Am I treating myself like a precious object?

Creative and constructive cooking requires good basic tools. There are different types of cookware that have advantages and disadvantages. You need to get rid of some of them as they are not good for you and put a strain on your digestion as you consume the leaching toxins. Your liver does a great job of detoxifying every day but can only cope with so much. A sluggish liver leads to sluggish digestion, bloating, constipation and even nausea.

Cooking vessels

Aluminium - These pans were used before stainless steel for many years. Acidic foods like oranges, tomatoes and vinegars and salty foods cause leaching of metals like aluminium as it is soft and highly reactive. Throw away anything that you eat off that is made with aluminium as it can leach into your food. Aluminium pans get thinner over time and where does it go? Into you! Some of you may be cooking roast dinners, or baked potatoes or fish in the oven wrapped in aluminium foil. Stop! It's harmful for you and your family. Instead, buy healthy baking paper from a health food shop or put your food in a glass casserole dish. The metal-food reaction with aluminium can produce aluminium salts that are absorbed into your body and are associated with impaired visual motor coordination, chronic inflammation in digestive disease and Alzheimer's.

Aluminium can build up in your body from various sources such as baking powder, salt, deodorant and antacids. Some people are more sensitive to aluminium than others especially if their digestive organs are not detoxifying it out of the body effectively. It will then build up in the fat cells and tissues of the body. Aluminium is the third most abundant element in the earth's crust and can be found in air, water and soil. It's best to take every opportunity to avoid exposure.

Anodised aluminium cookware - has become a popular alternative to plain aluminium. Aluminium placed in a chemical solution and exposed to electric current builds up a hard, non-reactive surface. This is called anodisation. The anodising process locks in the aluminium, but anodisation can break down over time.

Cast iron -This is considered good as these pans are heavy and thick and the heat distribution is more even, maintaining the cooking temperature uniformly. This prevents one part of the food from scorching or burning whilst another part is under heated. Raw cast iron pans are best treated with healthy oil before cooking. This fills in the porous surface of the cookware.

The best types are lined with enamel and care is needed when cleaning not to abrade the enamel surface. If this happens small amounts of cast iron can leach into the food. Ingesting small amounts of iron or iron oxide through cooking hasn't been shown to be dangerous to humans and some say it's of benefit. I'm a bit sceptical as iron from cookware is not organically derived and it's also non-chelated and therefore indigestible with no nutritional benefit. Cast iron is very easy to clean and lasts for generations.

Ceramic - Clay pots made from unglazed clay are generally healthy. The clay pot is usually soaked in water before cooking and during cooking. The pots help increase the tenderness and natural flavours of a dish. Pottery cookware has been used longer than cast iron. Originally cooking in India was done in ceramic pots over a bare flame. We don't have strict laws in Australia regarding coating on ceramic plates and bowls; especially those that come from China. Any pot or plate or bowl that is orange, yellow or red is likely to have cadmium or lead (heavy metals) in it. It is best to stick to white. If a ceramic dish or pot has a chalky or dusty residue after washing, discard it.

Copper - copper leaches into food when heated, causing the FDA to caution against using unlined copper pans for general use. The cooking surfaces of pans are usually lined with tin, nickel or stainless steel. Coated copper cookware can lose its protective layer if damaged or scoured. I find a lot of people we test have a high copper content in their body from water pipes and it causes many health problems; so avoiding it in pans is essential too. Bear in mind that the metals of the "protective" coating can also end up in your food.

Glass - lead-free glass cookware does not leach into food and is made from silica or sand. From this point of view it is the safest cookware. The only disadvantage of using glass cookware is its heat distribution inefficiency, the glass can break and there can be loss of nutrients due to the light from the heating element destroying light sensitive nutrients in food because of glass transparency; these are not affected by opaque cookware. Avoid using non-resistant glass cookware over heat as it can shatter. Glass cookware is not designed to go from the oven to the fridge and a change in temperature like this can cause it to shatter.

Stainless steel - this is safe and durable. Choose pots with heavy bases; preferably cooper bases as these distribute the heat evenly and steel is inert. This option is a mixture of different metals, including nickel, chromium and molybdenum. These metals can migrate into foods, but unless your cookware is worn or damaged the amount of metal likely to get into your food is not harmful.

As with non-stick pans, it is best to avoid using abrasives for cleaning stainless steel cookware.

Teflon coated vessels - I wouldn't recommend these as over time the teflon gets scratched off into the food and they have fluoropolymer coatings to prevent sticking. The fumes can also be toxic when cooking in these pans at high temperatures. According to the Environmental Working Group non-stick coatings can "reach 700° Fahrenheit in as little as 3-5 minutes, releasing 15 toxic gases and chemicals, including two carcinogens." At high heat the fluoropolymers used in non-stick finishes release various toxic substances and at least one greenhouse gas.

The biggest concern surrounds perfluorooctanic acid (PFOA), a substance that persists in the environment which is detectable in the blood of almost all Americans, adults and newborns. PFOA is considered a likely carcinogen and is associated with birth defects. It is known to cause testicular, pancreatic, mammary and liver tumours in rats. Workers exposed to PFOA have increased risk of pancreatic cancer and cancer of the male reproductive tract. These fumes have killed caged pet birds kept in kitchens. There is still research being done on its potential harmful effects. These pans are unfortunately very popular as they prevent food sticking. Never leave the stove unattended as toxicity becomes worse with overcooked or overheated food.

Titanium has many advantages due to beneficial titanium metal properties. It is usually healthier, lighter, lasts longer, heats quickly and is easy to clean. There can be confusion with non-stick titanium or titanium reinforced pans. Titanium can mean pure titanium material without any coating; while non-stick titanium or titanium reinforced pans often have coatings made of material similar to teflon. Titanium cookware that is safe is usually silver in colour. It is best to check with the manufacturer all the substances that go into the pan; some titanium pans are mixed with other metals. If they don't leach they are usually safe but the amount and types of metals will alter the quality of the pan.

Wok -These are good for stir fry's. Woks leave the factory coated with oil so it is important to wash them before use. Heat your wok with a thin coating of coconut oil or rice bran oil applied with a paper towel and let this heat for ten minutes allowing it to smoke. Repeat this once more as it prevents sticking. Slower cooking times with a wok may mean less nutrient damage. It is designed to cook food quickly so it is best to constantly stir it and avoid overheating the wok.

Safe chemical free cookware

There are some non-stick pans that have the coating baked on and these are a lot safer, like those that have a natural mineral base. Another safe alternative is one with a non-stick nano surface which is bonded at extreme temperature. Some of these pans have been certified by the Danish Institute of Technology as free from any emissions from PFOS, APFO and PFOA chemicals as found in most other non-stick cookware, such as gastrolux. There are also pans with an ecolon coating which is ecofriendly and totally chemical free, such as neoflam.

Environment - glass, ceramic and enamel cookware cannot be recycled. They can be used to serve multiple functions in the kitchen. Their longevity is limited by breakage.

Cooking methods

Baking - avoid using cooked foods that are not beneficial for you; for example, flaxseeds, which I have seen in breads for menopausal women, are not beneficial cooked as the molecules of the oil are too fragile and become harmful when cooked. Remember to use only the oils mentioned in "frying."

Barbeque - if wood coals are used there is a danger of undercooking some meats which allows some organisms to survive, especially if it's not thawed properly. There is a danger of cooking meats at high temperatures which causes the production of **Heterocyclic amines (HCAs)**. Research has shown that these are the carcinogenic chemicals formed when amino acids (from protein) and creatine (a chemical found in muscle) react at high temperatures e.g. with beef burgers, pork, fowl and fish. Researchers have identified 17 different HCAs resulting from the cooking of muscles in meats that may pose a risk of cancer. The consumption of meats that are burnt or barbequed are associated with colorectal, pancreatic and breasts cancers. People who eat medium-well or well done beef are more than three times likely to suffer stomach cancer than those who eat rare or medium-rare beef. On the contrary, cooking meat well helps destroy parasites but to be sure you avoid parasites it is ideal to freeze meat for 2 weeks and then you can have it rare.

High temperature cooking such as grilling and pan frying can still produce large amount of HCAs. So the message is cook and grill at low temperatures. Marinating meat before a barbeque is thought to reduce HCA production. If you like barbequing then precook your meat and add it to the barbeque for a short time to increase the flavour. Lemon juice added to meat several hours before cooking makes it much easier to digest and takes the pressure off your digestive system.

Another class of cancer causing substances are **Polycyclic Aromatic Hydrocarbons (PAH).** These are formed when meat drips onto coals and creates a smoke which deposits PAH onto meat. Trim the fat from the meat to prevent dripping onto flames and avoid all burnt positions.

Use low temperatures and slow cooking times. Consider casseroling and using a slow cooker.

Boiling - always add food to the boiling water, not beforehand. Most damage happens to water soluble nutrients especially vitamin C and B1, B12 and folate. The longer the time in the water the greater the nutrient loss e.g. blanching causes minimal nutrient loss. Left over water can be used for soups and stocks. Consider the heat, amount of water and time. It's better to add a small amount of water and let it absorb.

Frying - use low temperatures and only cook with butter, ghee, coconut oil or rice bran oil.

Grilling - use low temperatures; it's a good way not to have to use oil. Using baking paper from a health food shop on the grill tray prevents time washing up.

Microwave - Get rid of your microwave or only use it for heating wheat packs. It's used for expedience by many people and is quicker than conventional cooking. Since 1971 standards for safety and leakage have improved but it's not the way to go. Food molecules are bombarded by electromagnetic waves causing friction and heat. Nutrient damage occurs and there is a big concern with plastics coming into contact with food and the risk of Polyethylene Terephthalate (PET) being consumed. Metal put into microwaves can create toxic fumes. Please never consider microwaving breast milk. It loses lysosyme (an enzyme with antiseptic action) antibodies (which are essential for immunity) and can foster the growth of pathogenic bacteria.

Pressure cooking - using water and steam inside a sealed pressurised vessel, this reduces cooking time dramatically. It is excellent for legumes and softens and tenderises fibres. Studies have been done that show pressure cooking has the least negative affect on losing nutrients in cooking than boiling. Fewer water soluble nutrients are lost than through boiling.

Steaming - uses very little water and the nutrient loss is far less than boiling. Food is suspended in bamboo or a stainless steel basket over water.

Stir-frying - is good because it is quick and seals in moisture, so there is less nutrient loss. Water or coconut oil can be used.

When you eat out think twice about what your food has been through; consider bain-maries used at fast food outlets where the food sits for hours exposed to heat and light. There is a lot of nutrient loss. A lot of restaurants still use aluminium pans.

Antioxidants

The *Journal of the Science of Food and Agriculture* published a study done on the effects of antioxidants in different methods of cooking; it showed there was a reduction of antioxidants in all methods of cooking in varying amounts.

Microwaving 74-79% loss

Boiling 66% loss

Pressure cooking 47% loss

So it is therefore best to cook in stainless steel, ceramic or glass pans and to cook at low temperatures to conserve nutrition. To save time and enhance flavours in a dish consider a slow cooker/crockpot.

CHAPTER 5

The good, the bad and the ugly bugs

*"A wise man should consider that
health is the greatest of human
blessings and learn how, by his own thoughts,
to derive benefit from his illnesses."*

Hippocrates
(460 B.C.-377 B.C.)

CHAPTER 5
The good, the bad and the ugly bugs

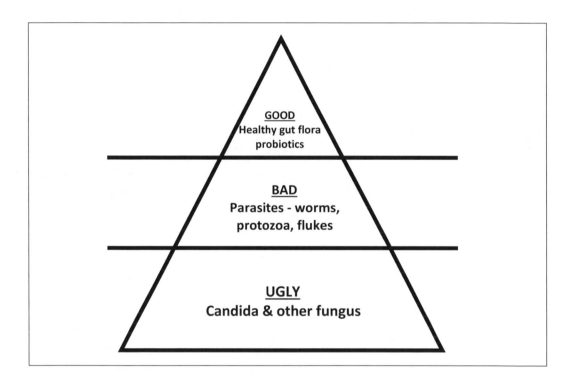

Several hundred species of good bacteria populate the large intestine which is about 165cm long. There are also beneficial bacteria throughout the small intestine and the good bacteria account for 30-50% of the volume of your poo! When this healthy balance gets disrupted by bad bacteria, often from an unhealthy diet, illness can develop and you also develop a lovely terrain for parasites and fungus to grow in. A lack of good bugs or an increase of bad bugs can alter the biochemistry of the brain causing behavioural disturbances in babies, children and adults.

Putrefactive matter in the intestine contains toxins, which can initiate violent inflammatory reactions that can produce carcinogenic substances in the intestine; however, good bugs can beneficially alter the course of disease. Live beneficial micro-organisms, the good bugs, are known as probiotics. Some probiotics produce B vitamins which have a profound effect on healthy nerves. Prebiotics stimulate the growth and activity of the healthy probiotics. Prebiotic foods that are beneficial are: Jerusalem artichoke, asparagus, chicory root, dandelion greens, onion, garlic, leek, unrefined barley and yacon syrup. For probiotics in fermented foods see chapter 9.

Bad bugs - what are they and where do they come from?

A healthy gut has an abundance of good bacteria which help stop parasitic infections. Bad bugs can be really detrimental to your health and unfortunately these parasites are on the increase and there are many of them. Sometimes parasitic infestations are undiagnosed and you may feel like a leech is sucking your energy from you, yet you are not aware you have them.

You may have heard of people venturing to Asia and getting a parasite or watched T.V. programs about Africans with parasites and thought there's no way I could ever have that. Parasites and worms are actually becoming more and more common with modern-day living. Generally Asian and African cultures have adapted their immune systems so they are not so susceptible to the parasites around them.

A parasite is an organism that can live off and reproduce in you. Parasites can survive for years in the human body and not only invade the intestines but penetrate your organs, lymph and even your brain! They can also be transferred from person to person and through food and contaminated water which are the most common sources. Parasites can be very depleting. They cause lethargy as they take vital nutrients from you and produce toxins which require energy for your elimination organs to deal with. They are more common than people think and are particularly common in people with chronic fatigue, candida albicans, autoimmune disease and cancers. Often parasites have been a contributing factor to these illnesses. There is the case of a lady who had bowel cancer and a large population of a parasite called 'blastocystis hominus' in her gut. The doctors could not eradicate this parasite but once they had removed the cancer from her bowel it vanished!

They are also nasty because they play havoc with your good bacteria and open you up to other health problems.

Parasites can cause a variety of symptoms or no symptoms at all. Usually the first symptoms are abdominal symptoms like tummy pain, gas, diarrhoea and bloating. A professional diagnosis is best to treat them. It is important to get a 3 day stool test from a reputable laboratory. Many stool tests from your doctor only involve 1 or 2 samples which aren't enough. If the parasites are in your organs usually a machine like a Mora machine is needed to diagnose where they are in the body as well as what they are.

What can make you more susceptible to parasites?

- Poor diet

- Poor gut health

- Leaky gut

- Lowered immunity

- Stress

- Travel

- Poor hygiene

- Exposure to infected people or pets

- Contaminated food and water

- History of antibiotic use

- Children in childcare

- Excessive consumption of undercooked meat or raw fish

- Unwashed vegetables contaminated with parasite eggs

- Low stomach acids and digestive juices

- Low bowel flora

- Walking barefoot on contaminated soil

How many parasites are there?

There are hundreds of parasites that can invade and exist in the human body. They can cause inflammation and immune problems. They can range in size from microscopic and unseen up to 10 metre long tapeworms! Some of these parasites can live within your body for most of your life. Your body tries very hard to adapt to their toxins and the waste that is excreted by them.

Signs and symptoms

Gut symptoms: This is the main site of parasitic infections and symptoms can include: chronic constipation, gas and bloating, very explosive bowel movements, diarrhoea, tummy pain, mucus in your stools, leaky gut, nausea, burping, weight loss, vomiting, burning in the tummy from inflammation, bloody stools, itchy anus, yeast infections like candida, food allergies, excessive saliva, bad breath, bad taste in the mouth and tummy cramping.

Allergy: Parasites can irritate and sometimes perforate the intestinal lining, allowing undigested molecules to leak through the bowel wall. This can activate the body's immune response which can inflame body tissue and then result in an allergic reaction.

Tiredness: The toxic waste overloads and overworks the organs and tires out the nervous system which causes chronic tiredness, dark circles under the eyes, lethargy and weakness in the body.

Skin problems: Inflammation from parasites can cause itching, sores, swelling and skin rashes. You can also be prone to pimples as the liver gets overloaded and the skin tries to eliminate toxins. Hives and other allergies can develop. You can experience a crawling feeling under the skin.

Hair problems: Dry hair, brittle hair and hair loss can occur as the parasite robs your body of precious nutrition.

Moods: Having something nasty in you, reproducing and giving off toxic waste is bound to change your mood. They can attack the nervous system and cause anxiety, lack of focus, depression and restlessness.

Sleeping problems: Being a nuisance to the body you can react to parasites during periods of rest, this in turn produces insomnia, teeth grinding during sleep, bed wetting, drooling whilst asleep, nightmares, frequently waking and disturbed sleep.

Weight and appetite problems: Parasites can choose what nutrition they like and rob you of what you need. Depending on the type of parasitic infestation, you can be underweight or overweight and malnourished. You can also have an excessive appetite.

Muscle and joint problems: Parasites can travel to almost all soft tissue including your joints and muscles where they cause cysts and inflammation. The toxins from parasites can then cause inflammation in the joints and muscles causing pain, cramping, numbness of the hands and or feet and chest pain.

Blood problems: As the parasites suck the nutrients out of you this can lead to anaemia as iron stores are lost.

Blood sugar imbalances: You can be prone to hypoglycaemia as blood sugar can drop which can make you weak and dizzy.

Infertility: As the immune system gets weak and the toxic waste invades the body you can get hormonal disruption, erectile dysfunction, cysts and water retention.

Immune problems These can manifest as viruses or bacteria that won't go away, sores that won't heal, respiratory problems and fever.

Granulomas: Granulomas are tumour-like masses that encase destroyed or large parasitic eggs. They develop most often in the colon or rectal walls but can also be found in the lungs, liver, peritoneum and uterus. They are a type of inflammation and develop from a collection of immune cells that wall off to protect the body from infestation.

Other conditions might also be tell-tale signs of a parasitic invasion like asthma, diabetes, epilepsy, acne, migraines, poor vision, body odour and even the biggest killers; heart disease and cancer.

It is important to get an accurate diagnosis as these signs and symptoms can represent other problems in the body unrelated to parasites.

The most common parasites in humans are protozoa, worms and flukes.

Protozoa are single celled parasites that can cause serious illness as they take over the intestinal tract. Some protozoa produce a cyst, which means they can be transported through food and water from one person to another. When they are in this cyst state they cannot be destroyed by digestive juices. Common protozoa that can cause illness are: giardia, entamoeba, cryptosporidium, blastocystis hominus, trichomonas vaginalis and toxoplasma.

Some protozoa

Giardia is microscopic, travels through the blood stream and can affect the whole body. It is protected by an outer shell that allows its survival outside the body and in the environment for long periods of time.

Most people become infected through food and water sources like tap water, streams or rivers. Giardia is also commonly transferred from a pet and by poor hygiene habits.

Blastocystis hominus is a very persistent parasite that seems to be on the increase and it's a more difficult one to treat. At low levels it can live in your intestines for years with no symptoms. When you are under stress, have a compromised immune system such as a virus or bacterial infection it can flare up and increase in numbers. Often it is not diagnosed properly and thought to be irritable bowel, allergies or stress. When it flares up, the symptoms can be relentless and include diarrhoea, bloating, abdominal cramping, excess wind, dark circles under the eyes, itching anus and exhaustion.

It is one of the hardest parasites to get rid of and usually needs professional naturopathic attention.

Toxoplasmosis usually occurs through raw or rare meat. It is one of the most common infections around the world.

Worms (nematoda) are multicellular parasites that often don't cause symptoms unless the infestation becomes severe. Common worms are roundworm, hookworm and pinworm.

Common worms

Nematoda (pinworms, hookworms and roundworms) easily travel around the body infecting organs.

Pinworms are tiny little white worms that wiggle when they come out. They are about 3/4 of an inch long and live in the intestine. At least 1 in 5 children get pinworms. They cause anal itching.

Hookworms are grey, curved and about 6 inches long. They come to a point at both ends and are shaped like a fishhook. One quarter of the world's population has hookworms, and one expert thinks that 50% of Americans have them. They are usually found in tropical areas where the soil is warm and moist. They lay eggs or larvae and usually incubate in soil. Hookworms burrow into the skin usually through the soles of the feet.

They can live inside the human body for up to 15 years!

Hookworms are the only worms with teeth. They often cause anaemia and are responsible for low birth weight and retarded growth of children as they suck the protein nutrients out of the blood of the mother, depriving the foetus. Unless you have a large infestation there are few visible symptoms apart from anaemia or pale looking skin and loss of energy. This makes the hookworm especially dangerous as it may go undetected.

Roundworms can vary in length from a centimetre up to a metre. Mature female worms have been estimated to produce an average of 200 000 eggs per day. They are common in tropical climates. Often there are no symptoms until a worm comes out of the anus, mouth or nostril! Ascaris are the most common. They can be up to 40 cm in length and often cause eczema in children.

In large numbers they can obstruct the bowels and there is one documented case where on autopsy of a two year old South African child was found to have over 800 giant roundworms weighing 19 ounces inside of her intestines. She had internal gangrene. Unfortunately you can get roundworms from your dog or cats. Experts have projected that at least half of these pets are infected with parasites. Think about that next time your dog gives you a loving kiss. Regularly deworm your pets as well as yourself.

Tapeworms (cestoda)

These parasites have been known to grow from an inch to 36 inches long and even longer. They can survive up to 25 years in the body.

Pork tapeworm taeniasolium from eating undercooked pork.

Fish tapeworm diphyllobothriumlactum from eating raw freshwater fish.

Tapeworm hymenoplepis from eating material contaminated by flour beetles and cockroaches.

Flukes (trematoda) are flattened oval or worm-like animals, usually no more than a few centimetres in length, although they can be as short as 1 millimetre or as long as 7 centimetres. Their main external feature is the presence of two suckers, one close to the mouth and the other on the underneath of the animal. They can be found anywhere where human waste is used as fertiliser and are most common in Asia. Schistosomiasis, which is also known as bilharzia, bilharziosis or snail fever is an example of a parasitic disease caused by one of the species of trematodes; platyhelminth infection, or "flukes."

Common trematoda - flukes

Lacer liver fluke dicrocoelium denriticum from ingesting ants

Liver fluke - fasciolosis from fresh water snails

Fasciolopsiasis - intestinal fluke from eating infested water plants or drinking infected water

Metagonimiasis - intestinal fluke from eating of undercooked or salted fish (freeze fish to avoid tapeworm)

Paragonimiasis - lung fluke from eating raw or undercooked freshwater crabs, crayfish or other crustaceans

How to prevent them

It's important to wash your hands before eating. What you touched might have parasites on it. Faecal contamination is another problem. Many times, human intestinal parasites are transmitted to another person via faecal contamination of water and foods. It's particularly true in less developed countries.

An extra precaution is to wash all vegetables and fruits especially before eating them raw. Because most vegetable growers use fertiliser they run the risk of contamination by faecal matter infested with human intestinal parasites.

They are commonly contracted from pets especially when your immune system is low.

Unwashed foods and raw animal products can contain parasite eggs so freeze meat for 2 weeks to destroy parasites.

If you have a vulnerable digestive system you can get parasites by walking barefoot in moist warm climates.

Pay attention to hygiene especially around infected people. Do not share towels, bars of soap, toothbrushes or kitchen utensils.

Avoid acidity and maintain a healthy pH.

If you feel you have a weak immune system wash your hands after shaking hands with people, without becoming obsessed!

Managing parasites

Eat fresh whole foods and keep carbohydrates low.

Avoid refined and processed food, sugar, soft drinks, caffeine, dairy and fruit juice.

Avoid damp food like dairy, sugar and wheat.

Increase intestinal flora (see Ch.9).

Strengthen digestion and immunity (see Ch.11).

If you have diarrhoea drink the liquid after cooking white rice.

Minimise stress.

Wash sheets and bedclothes every day whilst infected. This can be exhausting but is short lived.

Avoid sharing utensils and any other personal household items.

Consume protein at every meal.

Food is best cooked to minimise fermentation in the gut. Soups and stews with lots of garlic, turmeric and cloves. Miso broth and vegetable juices are also helpful.

Practice good hygiene.

Deworm pets.

Incorporate prebiotic food into your diet, this helps hold onto probiotics. Garlic, leeks, onions, artichokes and chicory root help.

Garlic in high doses is anti-parasitic. Use in cooking, in dips and spreads. Parsley takes away bad breath caused by garlic.

Adding cloves in your diet help kill eggs, pumpkin seeds and pawpaw seeds help kill parasites.

Citrus seed extract is very potent, powerful and has a strong taste. Take 4 drops in water 3 times a day. For herbal medicine see a naturopath.

Probiotic foods include fermented foods such as kefir, sauerkraut and plain yoghurt.

Solvents like benzene and propyl alcohol used in lotions and cleaning products help eggs to hatch faster. Without these, eggs pass through before they have time to hatch.

Drink filtered water.

Have colonic hydrotherapy/irrigation as part of your treatment plan.

Incorporate apple cider vinegar, lemon juice and bitter foods to help your upper digestion.

Under guidance, fasting on green vegetables, lemons and ginger can help starve them out.

Have you been on a very restrictive candida diet for months and are still not 100% well?

You may be harbouring a parasite or two or even a dozen! Parasites or worms are often the silent enemy hidden in your body. Please note, these symptoms can belong to another diagnosis so it is always best to get a professional diagnosis.

We use colonics and herbs and change the gut environment to kill parasites but diet is very important too! Here are some useful home remedies:

Food can be used to kill parasites:

1. Chew one handful of raw brown rice for breakfast – eat nothing else. Other meals during the day can be normal.

2. Between meals, eat 1 clove of garlic and 1 small handful of pumpkin seeds. Those who cannot tolerate raw garlic may slice the garlic and eat it between 2 slices of apple.

3. When 2 or more hours have passed since the last meal of the day, drink one cupful of mugwort tea (artemisia vulgaris).

4. Chew on a few cloves (the herb) until the taste has gone.

Follow this for 10 days, stop for 7, then resume for a final 10 to allow for any newly hatched eggs to die.

See pawpaw seeds in Ch 11 Kitchen Pharmacy.

It is most important to do this diet under the supervision of a health care practitioner to ensure optimum health.

Candida and other fungal infections

These can be nasty and persistent. They occur in 3 forms: yeast, mycelial and protoplast. They sometimes manifest as thrush in the genitals which can itch and produce a yeasty smelling discharge and or a thick white coasting on the tongue. Other signs include itchy red raised scaly patches on the skin. They often have sharply defined edges. Nails can become yellow, thick and crumble.

Risk factors

- Antibiotics

- The pill

- Steroids

- Imbalance of healthy flora and bacteria in the gut

- Leaky gut

- Excessive stress

- Excessive exercise

- Allergies

- Chemotherapy

- HIV/Aids

- Diabetes

- Low hydrochloric acid and enzymes

- Age - very young and old have more fragile immune systems

- Exposure to people or animals that have infections

- Poor hygiene

- Poor diet with excess sugar and yeast

Fungus likes heat and moisture, so if you sweat a lot you are more at risk. Wearing shoes and socks for prolonged periods and nail injuries can affect fungus in your nails.

Managing candida

If you have tried candida diets for many years and it comes back I'd highly recommend. The Specific Carbohydrate or GAPS diet. You will find a lot of information on this on the internet. It is also important to assess the immune system, adrenal glands, leaky gut, parasites, bowel flora, enzymes, hydrochloric acid and other fungal infections. Sometimes candida is just part of more complex health issues and often the liver is involved.

Diet

Avoid: sugar, soft drinks, fruit and fruit juices, yeast (breads, vinegar, mushroom processed meats, cheeses and vegemite), alcohol except gin and vodka.

Grains, especially wheat, potatoes, pumpkin are best avoided for 2 weeks then greatly reduced.

Include:

Fresh whole foods, natural yoghurt or kefir with live lactobacillus and cooked food that is easy to digest to avoid fermentation in the gut.

Include protein at every meal such as fish, eggs, meat, beans, lentils, chickpeas, seeds and nuts.

Increase garlic, onion, coconut oil, oregano, turmeric, olive oil and fresh vegetables.

Increase foods high in zinc like sunflower and pumpkin seeds.

Increase bitter and sour foods.

Drink Pau d'Arco tea.

Use 6 drops of tea tree oil and 2 drops of oregano oil in a bath. Add 3 drops of lavender oil if there is itching or burning.

Rest and minimise stress as much as possible to restore your immune system.

Wear natural fabrics and organic cotton or silk underwear if possible.

Keep skin clean and dry.

Avoid sharing personal items like towels, brushes or clothing.

Wear sandals at gyms, pools and wet areas.

Avoid touching infected pets.

If sexually active it is best that both partners address fungus to avoid reinfection.

When you have resolved your bad bugs keep up foods that help the gut lining like the fermented foods in Ch.9. Doing a detox can also be valuable see Ch.10. Often with a difficult journey of bug infestation you will have learnt to eat well, although it may have been challenging. Keep up the good habits and if you go off track your body will let you know if it's harmful for you.

CHAPTER 6

Easy and effective ways to eliminate constipation and help allergies

"Health is not valued till sickness comes."

Dr. Thomas Fuller
(1654-1734)

CHAPTER 6
Easy and effective ways to eliminate constipation and help allergies

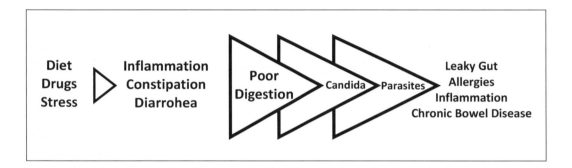

Allergies

We have got rid of many infectious diseases that ran rife in the human population in the past, however the modern world is a toxic world and with it, it has bought its own new plague.

One of your first lines of defence is your digestive system and for many this is becoming more and more damaged. Allergies are on the increase. In part, this reaction involves the gut as at least 70% of your immunity is in the gut.

Why are we becoming allergic to our planet?

The modern world has bought with it a new domestic environment and rapid modernisation has created the perfect storm to change your genetics. Over fifty years ago asthma hardly existed and now in modern world cities a shocking 1/3 of adults have asthma and 40% of children have asthma! It's astounding how toxic the air you breathe can be.

Amongst many families this is causing great distress. Peanut allergies, once never heard of, have caused deaths from anaphylactic shock and these deaths have doubled in the last 15years.

There is an amazing 700% increase in admission to hospitals in America for anaphylaxis from allergies. Strictly speaking, an allergy is immune mediated, quick and often dangerous whereas an intolerance involves a different immune response, it takes a longer time to react which can be anywhere from 6 hours to 3 days.

How did allergies increase?

Before the Second World War hardly any allergies existed but after the 1950s a lot more people started scratching, itching, wheezing and suffering from tummy troubles. More and more allergies occurred from latex to a multitude of food and environmental allergies. People's immune systems started to overreact to substances. Interestingly on an island in the Tristan da Cunha group in the south Atlantic every single family suffers from asthma.

Unfortunately, that means that half of the 266 inhabitants suffer from asthma. This is in part because they all descend from 7 people and 3 of those had asthma. Most people on the island are distant cousins. A scientist who spent 20 years studying these people found a gene that causes collagen to overproduce in the airway which causes an asthma attack but it is modern living and its toxic onslaught that adds to their suffering by making the gene express itself more often.

On the other side of the world allergy rates have trebled in the past few decades and the way in which we live has a big part to play. We have more stress, toxic buildings, more cars, more junk food, less raw food, less wholefood, more drugs, more vaccinations, more environmental toxins and more toxins on our skin with modern products. This is a big assault to our immunity and a challenge to our detoxification organs.

When people have moved from third world countries to modern cities, allergies and illnesses that never existed before often manifest themselves. For example, families that have moved from Mexico to California often have more asthma. Not surprisingly this is more common in those that live within 300 metres of a busy road or freeway. In Chinese medicine there is a direct link between the lungs and large intestine. A poor diet damages the intestinal lining giving rise to lung problems.

Professor Gilliland from the University of Southern California discovered that near busy roads particles in the air, invisible to the human eye are deposited into the lungs and they are covered with metals and other toxic elements. In clinical trials, subjects breathed in toxic particles which were equivalent to 40 hours of exposure near a busy road in California. It was found that the risk of allergic disease dramatically increased when near a major road and living in proximity to busy roads showed if someone would develop an allergic disease or not.

As a result of her research Dr. Barnes believes that people's health is worse in modern homes with off gassing from carpets, upholstery and building materials. It is not only this but modern processed foods disturbing and inflaming the gut, poor dietary habits, some drugs and an increase in cars and pollutants which makes it all much worse.

It's fascinating but not surprising that populations from rural Africa with no allergies, when moved to a modern setting develop allergies. In one group of people it was found that they had very high immunoglobulin E in their immune system. IGE is a class of antibodies (antibodies produced by the immune system to remove foreign particles from the body like toxins, viruses and bacteria) in the immune system that is very high in these Africans. IGE originally evolved as a protective mechanism against parasites and worms found in rural Africa. In modern countries IGE had no worms to bind to, so bound itself to innocuous substances like house dust for example.

So striving for modern luxury has a downside to the environment and that has a huge impact on your health. Many of you have become out of sync with the modern environment and so has the ecosystem in your gut.

Poor diets and some drugs like antibiotics can irritate the ecosystem of the gut and cause inflammation. This can lead to leaky gut (as explained in Ch.1) which can lead to food allergies.

You are all being poisoned to different degrees, so eating food as medicine, avoiding foods that are wrong for you, minimising the environmental overload of poisons and healing leaky gut (Ch.1) will ease your toxic burden and increase your health.

How to test allergies yourself

Whilst there are several machines and blood tests that show up allergies a simple one you can do for food allergies is the pulse test.

1. Get your baseline pulse by counting your pulse for a full minute before eating a food. Make sure you always test your pulse before and after the test sitting in the same position.

2. Put a food in your mouth on your tongue. Let it stay on your tongue, so that you can taste it for about two minutes. The taste will send a signal to your brain, which then sends a signal through the sympathetic nervous system to the rest of your body. It is best to test only one food at a time. Testing individual ingredients provides better information rather than testing foods containing several ingredients.

3. Retake your pulse while the food is still in your mouth. An increase of 10% or more may be considered an allergic/sensitivity reaction. The more allergic you are, the higher your pulse will be. Some foods may be borderline and worth eliminating.

4. Spit the food out and rinse your mouth out with some purified water, then spit the water out. Wait two minutes, then you can retest your pulse to see if it has returned to baseline. If it hasn't, wait 10 more minutes and retest until you have returned to your baseline pulse. You can then test the next food, repeating the procedure as frequently as you like, as long as your pulse returns to its baseline between tests.

If you experience an increased pulse rate, perform the test two more times to rule out other factors.

It is important that you are calm when you take your pulse as shock, noise, bright light and T.V. can increase adrenaline which raises your pulse rate and may give a false allergy reading.

Alternatively you can take foods you suspect you are sensitive to out of your diet for 3 weeks. Then bring them back one at a time leaving a 3 day gap between each food. You will get an exaggerated reaction of what that food is doing to your body over the 3 days. These symptoms can vary, for example headaches, mood changes, bloating, gas, nausea, excessive thirst, mood changes, skin problems, respiratory problems, muscle pain, irritable bowel and diarrhoea.

Once you find out what the offending foods are, take them out of your diet for 3 months to give your body a rest, then bring one back in a tiny amount. For example, if it's wheat, eat only a few crumbs of wheat a day. This usually stops an allergic reaction occurring and allows your immune system to get used to tolerating the food. If you react to tiny amounts (which can happen up to 72 hours after eating the food) take the food out for another 3 months otherwise continue having very small amounts of that food for a few weeks, then gradually increase the amount as your body tolerates it. In some cases where the gut lining needs a lot of repair the food may need to be eliminated from your diet for a couple of years.

The most common allergies are: dairy (often raw milk is okay), soy, citrus, peanuts, wheat, fish, eggs, corn, chocolate, sugar, tomatoes and food additives.

Fructose is such a common intolerance, tested through a hydrogen breath test and usually emerges from a tired pancreas. Sometimes people are not intolerant but it's just not good for them and causes insulin problems and weight gain. Agave, a natural sweetener, is high in fructose and fructose is a no no if you are overweight, trying to lose weight, have PCOS, Syndrome X, insulin resistance or diabetes. Even if you do not test allergic or intolerant to it, high fructose foods aren't recommended with these conditions.

Fructose is a monosaccharide (simple sugar), which the body can use for energy. Because it does not cause blood sugar to rise (has a low glycaemic index), it was once thought that fructose was a good substitute for sugar however, nutritional experts have changed their minds about this.

What happens if I consume too much fructose?

Most of the carbohydrates that we eat are made up of chains of glucose. When glucose enters the bloodstream, the body releases insulin to help regulate it. Fructose is processed by the liver and if the liver can't process it fast enough for the body to use as sugar, it starts making fats from the fructose and sending them off into the bloodstream as triglycerides which are a risk factor for heart disease.

Symptoms of fructose intolerance can include:

- Bloating

- Diarrhoea

- Gas

- Abdominal pain

- Mood swings

- Nausea

There is a problem with foods especially fruits high in fructose when the fructose content is higher than the glucose content. For a person without fructose intolerance it is not recommended to have more than 25-30mg of fructose per sitting. The most common diet for fructose intolerance is the FODMAP diet. Initially this is strict, then after 3 weeks various foods can be slowly added back. What I have found that does work is avoiding the foods below, doing a lot of work to strengthen the digestive system and working with foods and herbs to help improve the function of the pancreas and liver.

Foods to avoid (fructose is higher than glucose)

- Fruit - apple, pear, guava, honeydew melon, nashi fruit, mango, quince, star fruit, watermelon;

- Dried fruit — apple, currant, date, fig, pear, raisin, sultana;

- Fortified wines

- Foods containing added sugars such as agave syrup, honey, some corn syrups (check packets of foods and breads), and fruit juice concentrates.

- Onions

Favourable foods (fructose equal to or less than glucose)

The following list of favourable foods is from the paper: "Fructose Malabsorption and Symptoms of Irritable Bowel Syndrome Guidelines for Effective Dietary Management."

- Stone fruit: apricot, nectarine, peach, plum;

- Berry fruit: blueberry, blackberry, boysenberry, cranberry, raspberry, strawberry, loganberry;

- Citrus fruit: kumquat, grapefruit, lemon, lime, mandarin, orange, tangelo;

- Other fruits: ripe banana, jackfruit, kiwi fruit, passion fruit, pineapple, rhubarb, tamarillo.

Is fructose bad for me?

A small amount of fructose, such as the amount found in most vegetables and fruits, is not a bad thing however, consuming too much fructose at once seems to overwhelm the body's capacity to process it. The diets of our ancestors contained only very small amounts of fructose.

Pancreas

Fructose overwhelms the pancreas but sugar is worse. To strengthen the pancreas remove all sweet foods and include in your diet: fermented foods, ginger, fennel, dill, bitter melon, garlic, cardamom, cinnamon, apple cider vinegar and lemons. Your naturopath may need to test you for a deficiency of digestive enzymes which are important for pancreatic function.

Constipation

One of the most frequent bowel problems experienced today is constipation. A constipated system is slow to release toxic wastes and the compacted consistency of the stool makes it difficult to pass and causes strain. This can lead to haemorrhoids and other bowel problems. The longer waste is in your colon the more proteins can putrefy, fats can become rancid and carbohydrates can ferment into unfriendly bacteria. The longer your body is exposed to rotting food in your intestines, the greater the risk of developing disease. Even with one bowel movement a day you still have at least three meals making their journey down your lengthy digestive tract. As well as this, your system can also become self-polluting by the poisonous gases that are caused by stagnation in your bowel and unfriendly bacteria. These can enter your blood stream and cause inflammation in your body and irritate your liver. Alternating between constipation and diarrhoea can also mean there are unfriendly bacteria sitting inside you. Constipation can be linked to a hormonal imbalance, and hormones need to be excreted through the bowel after being metabolised by the liver.

On a more serious note, if you let a toxic bowel continue it can lead to cancer and immune dysfunction. If you have inadequate bowel movements you are creating a fertile breeding ground for serious disease.

Gastroenterologist, Dr. Anthony Bassler, tells his colleagues, "Every physician should realise that the intestinal toxaemias (poisons) are the most important primary and contributing causes of many disorders and diseases of the human body."

The large intestine is the body's "sewer system" and if you don't treat it well you can accumulate toxins which can lead to many different diseases.

Bowel movements are essential for good health. If you don't have at least one good movement a day you may be making your way towards disease. If you have a typical western diet you may hold 8 or more meals inside you whereas with a high fibre diet you usually hold only 3. Constipation can lead to leaky gut which is discussed more in Ch.7. Diet is a major part of treatment in healing the mucosa on the gut wall as food comes into contact with the gut mucosa.

Everyone benefits from a healthy bowel cleanse especially those that have parasites, a fungus, allergies or digestive problems.

So how often do you go to the toilet and how much? Many people think that constipation is not being able to go to the toilet for a few days and then having to strain to get it out. This is one type of constipation and can be very toxic to the body. You can imagine what happens if you leave food in your waste bin for several days it starts to rot and smell. This also happens in your digestive system and with meat it can be like dead or rotting flesh.

I am not opposed to people eating organic meat but if someone is prone to constipation it causes a lot of problems because as it rots it becomes very toxic. Generally too much animal protein can cause constipation and putrefaction. However, other foods and unnatural foods can also be toxic for example, preservatives, colouring, additives, refined foods and man-made drinks. It has been shown that people who emigrate and settle in another country can pick up a bowel disease that didn't exist in their culture because of a different diet that is unhealthy for them. This has been seen with Asians moving to America and islanders moving to Australia.

Constipation can be from the bowel being overly contracted and tight or being overly expanded and flaccid with weak muscles. It is usually caused by eating too much protein, fat, salt or white flour. The latter often happens from abusing laxatives, being chronically constipated, because of a lack of nutrients which strengthen the bowel, or from having too much fruit, juices or salads.

Please note: in some instances chronic constipation can result in liquid diarrhoea, which is waste material passing around solid stools that are blocking the colon.

If you are an adult and you are eating three meals a day then you should be passing the amount of stool each day from your wrist to your elbow in length. That may seem like an extraordinary amount for some but it may be that it is evacuated in several pieces (at least 10cm in size) and more than once a day. You want the diameter or width of your stool to be at least 2-3cm; this is about half the length of your thumb. Really thin stools indicate spasm of the bowel, or constipation or irritation of the bowel wall. Wide stools can be a problem if they overstretch the bowel and cause bleeding.

Now I know some of you are just passing rabbit stools or really small stools but there is hope. By the end of this book you will have lots of advice and if you follow it, your bowel movements will greatly improve. Constipation can also happen when someone eats too much psyllium (psyllium is positive for some types of constipation as long as you have enough water), dairy, fat or a lack of water or fibre.

The bowel relies on a wave-like action called peristalsis. It moves a bit like a caterpillar and this wave like action causes muscular contractions of the bowel/intestines. If you have too much heat or stagnation in your liver you will get dry, hard stools, often like balls, that are difficult to pass. If you have this type of constipation your tongue may be red with a thick coating at the back.

When the body is deficient or lacking in iron the strength of peristalsis is poor. Conversely, certain iron supplements can cause constipation.

You can be constipated even though you go to the toilet every day; you just don't go enough. If you want to test your transit time eat some corn kernels (it doesn't digest well) and then have a look in the toilet bowl for the next two days, when you open your bowels note when the sweet corn moves through. Ideally you don't want food staying in your bowels for more than 24 hours. You can do the same with beetroot. It's also a great bowel cleanser, full of iron and vitamin C which helps the absorption of iron.

Eating healthy nourishing foods supports the gut mucosa which is the lining of the gut wall. When you don't have enough fibre or you eat the wrong foods, take recreational drugs and certain medical drugs like antibiotics the gut wall becomes damaged which affects the absorption of nutrients and screening of harmful toxins. This can also lead to constipation.

Beware that chronic constipation puts a lot of stress on the heart and many people have had heart attacks on the toilet from persistent straining and pressure. I used to work in hospitals as a nurse and saw many problems caused by constipation. Recently a nurse told me about a sad case of severe constipation. A lady in her 60s came into casualty thinking she had a bowel obstruction. She was a nurse herself and had bowel problems for some time but neglected to address them. X-rays were taken which did not show an obstruction but severe constipation. Shortly after her X-rays were taken she had a heart attack as the pressure of constipation had put such a strain on her heart. The doctors tried to revive her but sadly she died but as they tried to revive her, faecal matter came through her mouth! A horrible story I know but this is the extreme of what can happen if you don't look after your bowels!

So what are the main causes of constipation and why do so many people have it?

Lack of water

Your body uses up a lot of water each day, breathing, sweating, digesting and carrying out metabolic activities in the body. The more salty foods you eat the more water your body requires. On average, you require 33mls of water per kg of body weight. So if you are only 48 kgs that's

1584 mls of water a day; in other words just over 1½ litres. On the other hand, if you are 100kgs you require 3300 mls of water a day or just over 3 litres so it is a lot more challenging if you are on the larger size.

If you don't drink enough water your intestines will not be able to move waste effectively and you'll get constipated. It is best to have filtered water systematically through the day having some every half hour to hydrate you well. Having nothing for hours and then a litre all at once can overtax the kidneys and cause you to pee out too many minerals. However, you are better to do this than let yourself go without and become dehydrated. Of course, if you are very active or living in a hot climate you will need even more water.

It is best to have the purest water you can afford but if good water is unavailable don't put off drinking. It's more important to drink tap water than nothing at all. Ideally, you should have water that has no heavy metals, chlorine or fluoride. Hot water or warm water is a lot easier to absorb.

Remember, water is water and energy drinks, soft drinks, tea and coffee don't count even though you may love them. Caffeine is a diuretic and causes you to urinate, so you won't retain the water you need, besides that, it makes you more acidic as a result of peeing out minerals.

If you find water boring, add half a lemon or lime. This will do wonders for your body. Even though lemons are acid outside the body they become alkaline inside the body. Lemon and lime will perk you up, help flush your lymph and liver and aid digestion.

Lack of fibre

Dietary fibre is the indigestible part of plant food. Today's diet lacks a lot of fibre and a variety of fibre is needed to prevent constipation and help move toxins. Fibre is largely indigestible so does not cause a gain in calories and therefore is also good for weight loss; in moderation it is very good for all round health. As well as preventing constipation, fibre prevents haemorrhoids, diverticular disease and is protective against polyps and cancer. With a high fibre diet there is less risk of heart disease, diabetes, high blood pressure, gall bladder problems and obesity.

There are 3 main types of fibre:

Insoluble fibre is also known as roughage and absorbs water and promotes bowel movements. This fibre resists digestion and is fermented by bacteria to produce special substances for the gut wall. It is found in the skins of vegetables and fruit, wheat bran, rice bran, dried beans, seeds and nuts. Wheat bran is often too abrasive and besides so many people are intolerant to gluten and Australian wheat. Out of all the vegetables, the green leafy ones usually have the most fibre, help the bowel by stimulating the liver and are high in minerals e.g. bok choy, kale, chard, silverbeet, spinach, rocket and endives. Animal food has no fibre; it is just found in plant food.

Soluble fibre is often slippery and holds lots of water forming a gel. It ferments in the colon and binds to fatty acids pulling out toxins, helps irritable bowel, cholesterol and regulates blood sugar. This includes oat bran, beans, some nuts, dried peas, lentils, barley, flaxseeds, slippery elm, apples and carrots. Chia seeds have both soluble and insoluble fibre. Soluble fibre is gentler on the gut than other fibres.

Resistant starch is found in whole grains, lentils, bananas and maize. It ferments in the gut and this has beneficial effects on the bowel wall and cholesterol.

Many people need a bulking grain to make them go to the loo. This can be brown rice, quinoa, buckwheat or millet. If you are really constipated then oat bran mixed with boiling water is excellent. If you can't eat bran from oats use rice bran. You can combine it with berries, yoghurt, or almond, rice or oat milk. Fruit with peel will also help the bowel move. Soaked prunes, flaxseeds, figs, plums, raw fruits and vegetables can also help. Plums and prunes have a lot of antioxidants and offer a lot of protection for your body. If you suffer from frequent bloating I would avoid fruit.

Remove white

If you suffer from constipation take out every white food e.g. white flour which includes breads, cakes and all things made with white flour, white pasta, yes even croissants and doughnuts! cheese, milk and white sugar.

Many of you will have a diet that is not nutrient dense and full of white and sugary foods such as sweets, cakes, ice-cream and lollies. Sweet drinks such as flavoured sodas and coke are also no good. These foods will fill you up but leave you malnourished. You can actually be fat and starving at the same time! Your body may just be getting energy from empty foods. These foods rob nutrients from the body and use up more nutrients trying to digest them than they contain. They are full of empty calories.

Avoid junk foods and bad oils (see Ch.8). The only oils to be cooked with are coconut oil, rice bran oil, ghee and butter and olive oil at a low temperature. Oils are useful for bowel movements but only healthy oils.

Top foods for your gut

For most people a variety of different fibres helps travelling stools. If there is persistent bacterial growth in your gut sometimes fibre needs to be avoided altogether for a while and a herbal laxative used if there is constipation. For these people, The Specific Carbohydrate Diet (SCD diet) or Gut And Psychology Diet (GAPS diet) can work well.

Foods that help constipation

In some cases, constipation responds better to no fibre and a healthy wholefood diet with good oils and green vegetables.

- Foods that lubricate the intestines and soothe inflammation: virgin olive oil, flaxseed oil, plain yoghurt and slippery elm bark.

- Foods that help intestinal flora: kefir, plain yoghurt, sauerkraut and fermented foods (Ch.9)

- Foods that help move the bowel: whole grains like brown rice, quinoa, buckwheat and millet. Figs, green leafy vegetables, oat bran mixed with hot water, rice bran, ground linseeds, chia seeds, kuzu, prunes, agar agar and psyllium husks.

- Often constipation is due to stagnation in the liver and a lack of bile flow. Bitter and sour foods, a low saturated fat diet and dandelion root help.

Teas for movement

Some herbal teas will hydrate you but some, like dandelion root, are diuretic. So whilst this tea is excellent for the liver and constipation you still need water. Dandelion root tea works really well for constipation in moderate doses. I like the bitter taste but some people don't. To change the taste, add a peppermint teabag. You can also have dandelion root with any type of milk (it's nice in chai) and a little bit of rice syrup. Other teas that help are senna leaf, rhubarb root, cascara sagrada bark, barberry bark, chamomile, liquorice root and ginger. Chamomile and liquorice are also anti-inflammatory.

Agar Agar

This is a translucent gel from red algae, rather like gelatine. It can be used to move the bowel and for obesity as it helps you feel full. You add it to hot water until it dissolves and then put it in the fridge until it goes like jelly. During the process you can add goji berries or other fruits for a sweet treat. It can also be used as a thickener in soups and it helps remove toxic and radioactive waste from the body.

Source - It is easy to get from Chinese and health shops. Keep in a cupboard in a sealed container.

Gelatine

This food may sound gross to some but I can't say enough about how healing this is for the intestines. It helps lubricate the intestines but more importantly it heals leaky gut and provides valuable nutrients for the gut. I have seen amazing health results with this food. See Ch.11 for bone broth recipe.

Flaxseeds

Flaxseeds are anti-inflammatory, laxative, hormonal balancing and they have an anti-platelet action, in other words they help thin the blood.

Flaxseeds are an exceptional source of fibre containing both soluble and insoluble fibre which is gentle on the gut. Bowel movements are improved and become more regular. This is partly due to the high amount of magnesium in flaxseeds which causes the bowel muscle to relax, then moves matter along an easier passage. Magnesium also relaxes the nervous system, so if you get constipated because you are tense this helps too.

Flaxseeds contain a substance called lignan and have one of the highest lignan contents of any vegetable or plant. This woody substance converts, with the assistance of bowel flora, to hormone-like agents which have been shown to have a protective effect against breast cancer. By helping the bowels you are helping prevent many other problems in the rest of your body. As mentioned, a sluggish bowel can also give rise to heart disease and studies have shown a 10% decrease in heart disease as a result of eating flaxseeds over several years. Obviously the whole diet and lifestyle are an adjunct to this.

Other hormonal problems can be exacerbated by constipation. Both the fibre aspect of flaxseed and the oestrogen regulating effect can also be applied to irregular cycles and menopause.

Source and storage

You can use flaxseeds whole (better for inflammation) or ground (better for fibre). You can buy ground linseeds or grind them yourself; these are best bought organic from a fridge.

Store them in a fridge or freezer when you get home. You can add a tablespoon of flaxseeds to porridge or salad. Ideally it is best to grind them at home in a food processor or coffee grinder for maximum freshness. Ground flaxseeds are unstable and affected by light and air. If you are buying the oil, only buy it in dark bottles with added vitamin E. The oil should taste sweet and nutty not rancid. Flaxseeds are a great addition to yoghurt and kefir but not for cooking as they are not stable when heated.

Rice bran

This is high in antioxidants and has high levels of vitamin E. It is also very high in fibre and is gentle on the gut. It contains something called Gamma Oryzanol which acts as an antioxidant and can reduce cholesterol oxidation. Cholesterol only tends to be a problem when it oxidises.

When bran is removed from grains, the grains lose a large portion of their nutritional value. Rice bran also contains a high level of dietary fibres known as beta-glucan, pectin and gum.

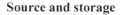

Source and storage

You can buy rice bran from a health food shop.

Store in a glass or ceramic container in a dark cupboard. You can add rice bran to any flour recipe for example, breads and muffins. You can also add a tablespoon to porridge or yoghurt.

Figs

The fruit that is highest in fibre is the fig and it is also very high in calcium. These can be eaten alone or with nuts or added to oat bran. If you have blood sugar issues minimise fruit and eat it with nuts or coconut oil. Figs may cause problems if you have a fructose intolerance.

Source and storage

Dried figs can be bought all year round and can be sourced organically from health food shops.

Store in a glass jar. Fresh figs grow in warm climates.

Chia seeds

Sprinkle onto porridge, soups or salads. They are a wonderful source of fibre and become jellylike when wet. For more detail see Ch.8 and Ch.12 for recipes. For extra fibre you can grind them in a blender.

Source and storage

They are found in health food shops and can be stored in a glass jar.

Psyllium husks

These are a gentle soluble fibre with a natural mucilaginous bulk forming agent which absorbs water to form a soft and bulky mass that makes bowel movements easier. Psyllium also pulls out excess cholesterol and toxins from the gut. It is not retained in the body and moves through you like a gentle broom. Incidentally if you take it with lots of water it helps constipation but if you take it with a little water it helps colitis and other conditions where there is diarrhoea. In this incidence it will slow the bowel down and help the awful feeling of not wanting to go out if there's a lack of public toilets. If you are constipated and don't use enough water with psyllium or you have very weak bowel muscles there is a danger of constipation. For constipation add one teaspoon to a large glass of water and drink immediately or mix it with yoghurt or breakfast food. Psyllium can also be added to baked goods like healthy muffins.

Tips: Other uses include gluten-free baking, where ground psyllium seed husks bind the moisture and help make breads less crumbly.

Source and storage

They are found in health food shops, supermarkets and Indian food shops. Store in a container below 30°C.

Kudzu

This is a wonderful root you can get from a health food shop. It's small and white and it helps get rid of dryness in the body and allows you to have a bowel movement with ease. You can mix a teaspoon in cold water and drink it or you can use it in cooking as a gelling agent. It is a healthier alternative to corn starch and potato starch as these are highly processed. Kudzu also regulates blood sugar and boosts immunity. Interestingly, it's had recent press for helping alcoholism. I use it for most digestive problems as it also helps with bloating, wind and ulcers.

Recipe: Dissolve 1tbsp. of kudzu in a cup of water and cook it until it is thick. For taste add a few sprinkles of tamari, you can also add some umeboshi paste and grated ginger for extra digestive support.

Olive oil

Taking two tablespoons of extra virgin organic olive oil before bed lubricates the bowel, easing constipation.

Slippery elm

It soothes the gut lining allowing it to heal and is a mild laxative.

Lack of exercise

One of the best ways to start the day and get the bowel moving is with a brisk walk in the morning. Go on, set that alarm half an hour earlier and just jump out of bed without thinking! Put on your tracksuit and get moving. You'll feel better for the whole day by doing it. If you find it difficult in the winter, get up five minutes earlier have a warm cup of lemon water or herbal tea and get one of your neighbours to walk with you. It's always easier with company. If you like pets and don't have your own, you could even offer to take a neighbour's dog out for a brisk walk. You'll be amazed at how many people are out and about in the early mornings with or without their dogs, in parks and on ovals; it becomes quite a friendly community.

Any type of exercise will help and if you have up to two hours a day to walk it will make a huge difference but even fifteen minutes is good. Deep breathing will help even more if you can do it during exercise. You were designed to move. Primitive societies may walk up to 40km a day just to gather food. Regular exercise also reduces inflammation and prevents obesity. Other exercises you can do are swimming, running, dancing, bicycle rides and gym work. Walking avoids injury that overdoing other exercises cause.

Interestingly, no animal runs for more than three minutes at a time in its natural environment. If you've watched wildlife shows you've probably seen lions chase zebras or other animals. The lion is running for lunch and the zebra is running for their life and the chase is brief. If the lion is not successful in a short time it stops and looks for a slower moving food source. The chase does not go on for miles and animals usually do not suffer from running injuries. You can always increase the pace of your walking and whatever exercise you choose it's important that you enjoy it and that it is injury free.

Your body needs to move and ideally in fresh air. Moving the body not only helps your circulation and fitness, it also helps your bowels to move. All exercise is good, in particular a rebounder or lymphaciser is ideal for bowel health (and great for the lymphatics). High quality lymphacisers are available from info@detoxspecialist.com.au. They have superior springs and are built to last for many years. They are also strong enough to take 105kg of weight.

Stress

It cannot be emphasised enough how much stress plays a part in digestion and bowel function. Have you ever been nervous before an exam and felt it in your tummy? Have you ever been so struck with fear that your bowels seem to freeze? Have you got so nervous before a driving test and can't get off the toilet as you have constant diarrhoea? Most of you have had the experience of getting a fright, feeling terrified or excited and it affecting your gut. You may have experienced diarrhoea, nausea or butterflies.

There is a direct link between the brain and the gut and chronic stress can lead to all sorts of gut issues including irritable bowel, ulcers and inflammatory bowel disease.

There are different types of stress and one type of stress produces a lot of adrenaline which gives you diarrhoea before an event like taking an exam. Other stress causes your body to contract and your bowel muscles to hold on. Find someone to talk to about your stress or get professional help. Take half an hour every day to do something that really relaxes you. This could be exercise, music, art, gardening or meditation.

Constipation itself has a big effect on mood. I'm sure you've noticed how much better you feel when you have a good movement every day! Often worrying about the future causes more bowel movement and anxiety. Being stuck in the past causes more constipation and depression.

Exhaustion often begins in the gut. The gut is the main source of nourishment for the rest of your body. Your digestion and assimilation need energy to function. If your energy, chi or prana are low then absorption suffers and consequently energy is reduced. The average diet in the western world taxes our digestive system over time. The nerves to the bowel get affected by stress and nutrient absorption may become suboptimal and then there is even less resistance to stress further leading to poor bowel function.

Along with dietary changes, look at getting help for emotional pain and stress. There are many good therapists out there and I can recommend E.F.T. and N.E.T. and hypnotherapy as well as traditional therapists.

You can get so used to being stressed you don't realise the impact it has. To help, start to add things to your life that ease your stress. There is lot of evidence that meditation has a huge impact on stress.

Community helps stress

Interestingly, a large group of people migrated from a town called Rosseto in Italy to New York. Here they created a mini Rosseto. What was curious about them was that they were happy, had no peptic ulcers, no bowel disease, hardly any heart disease, no suicide and no drug addiction. A lot of them were obese and didn't have good diets. Their health success came from a powerful and supportive social structure that cared about their people.

In "Risk Factor for Serious Illness" Vanitallie says, "In modern society, which is characterised by a rapid pace of life, high demands, efficiency and competitiveness in a global economy, it is likely that lack of rest, recovery and restitution is a greater health problem than the absolute level of stress."

Those that have regular relaxation in their life have less impact on their health when sudden shocks hit them.

15 tips on how to cultivate contentment

1. Nourish a garden

2. Create meaningful relationships

3. Appreciate what you have

4. Have a sense of purpose and meaningful goals

5. Live in the moment

6. Bring up a child

7. Cultivate optimism

8. Practice relaxation

9. Spend time in nature

10. Exercise for 30 minutes a day (high intensity exercise is good for anxiety)

11. Avoid junk food

12. Eat well - have a low sugar Mediterranean diet

13. Sleep well

14. Avoid addictions like alcohol, sugar, drugs and cigarettes

15. Nod your head to remember things positively

20 great stress reducers

1. Music

2. Dancing

3. Painting

4. Singing

5. Massages

6. Hugging

7. Laughing

8. Meditation

9. Writing a journal

10. Being in nature/watching a sunset

11. Breathing slowly and deeply

12. Set priorities

13. Forgive others

14. Control only what you can control

15. Keep things in perspective

16. Avoid dwelling on things

17. Use visualisation

18. Manage finances

19. Develop communication skills

20. Use lists

Useful apps for your phone:

Relax and Rest by Meditation Oasis

Mnf- Mindfulness Meditation by Mental Workout Inc.

At Ease - Anxiety and Worry Relief by Meditation Oasis

Nature Space - 3D Sound Holographic Audio Theatre.

Useful websites

For more information to relieve stress go to www.freemeditation.com.au, www.beyondthemind.com and www.researchingmeditation.com

For family mental health www.copmi.net.au

The following is a simple but very effective meditation used by Dr. Ramesh in his meditation research program at the University of Sydney. I have used this successfully on clients in my clinic and it has been a useful tool to enhance their lives.

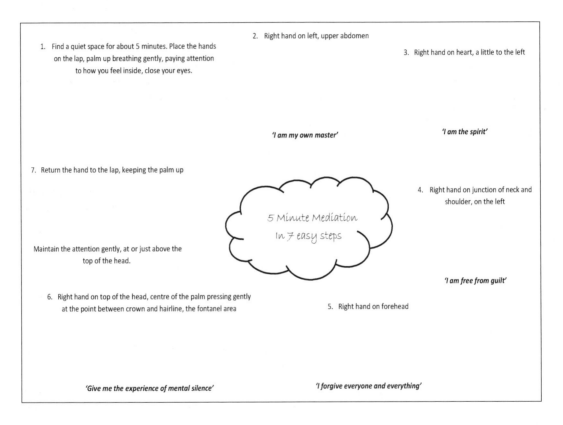

1. Find a quiet space for about 5 minutes. Place the hands on the lap, palm up breathing gently, paying attention to how you feel inside, close your eyes.

2. Right hand on left, upper abdomen

3. Right hand on heart, a little to the left

'I am my own master'

'I am the spirit'

7. Return the hand to the lap, keeping the palm up

4. Right hand on junction of neck and shoulder, on the left

5 Minute Mediation
In 7 easy steps

Maintain the attention gently, at or just above the top of the head.

'I am free from guilt'

6. Right hand on top of the head, centre of the palm pressing gently at the point between crown and hairline, the fontanel area

5. Right hand on forehead

'Give me the experience of mental silence'

'I forgive everyone and everything'

Other tips:

Chew well

It is really important to chew your food well. When you chew well your food is coated in enzymes produced by your saliva and is pre-digested, this helps the small intestine absorb nutrients and helps strengthen the pancreas which will then produce more enzymes to help you digest.

Blood building

If you are very deficient and thin your blood may need building and strengthening in order to help the bowel. In this case eating rice, millet, seaweed, beetroot and black beans helps. If you are anaemic you will need to build iron with red meat or beetroot, algae, seaweed, spirulina, dark leafy greens and apricots. It is essential to have enough vitamin C to absorb iron. Whilst beetroot has vitamin C, meat does not. People who are deficient and weak often lack B vitamins found in whole grains. As you become more nourished you will absorb more vitamins and minerals from your food. This will then build you up and strengthen your intestines.

Other causes of constipation

Neglecting the call of nature causes stagnation, so it is best to train your bowel by sitting on the toilet at the same time every day for 10 minutes, if you have constipation. Some people get into terrible habits by feeling they are too busy to go to the toilet, drink water or eat healthy food. If this is you, have a look at your priorities. It's important that you are healthy so you can be effective.

Habitual use of laxatives and a lack of potassium can cause constipation.

Please note: certain illnesses like hypothyroid, liver dysfunction and tumours can cause constipation. Tests from your doctor or naturopath are sometimes essential to determine the cause.

Nasty stories - There have been several cases of people dying from constipation due to bowel perforation. A few years ago in Ballarat, Victoria a teenage boy hadn't had his bowels open for six weeks. He virtually lived on fast food. After the six weeks he went to hospital and was flown to Melbourne for emergency surgery but sadly didn't make it due to peritonitis and blood poisoning after a perforated bowel.

Please look after your bowel now. What's one thing you can do today to make a difference to your bowel?

Enemas help constipation (for coffee enemas see Ch.10) - They can be used to help clear the bowel and introduce herbs and clays rectally. You can buy enema kits that you fill with 2 litres of pure warm water to clear your lower bowel. (available from info@detoxspecialist.com.au www.

detoxspecialist.com.au) You will get instructions with the kit. You can add different things into the water for varying effects (see the end of Ch.10).

Colonic hydrotherapy (closed method) can have a profound effect on constipation. It uses many litres of water and is much more effective than an enema. As well as waste being eliminated, the bowel wall is strengthened and the treatment is gentle. (see Ch.10).

Castor oil and Epsom salts

If you are really constipated, castor oil or epsom salts will help orally but beware they are strong and you want to be at home the morning after you take it! This shouldn't be done frequently as they are depleting.

Castor oil packs

This remarkable oil has been shown to deeply penetrate internal organs when used as a pack. See Ch.10 for how to use them.

Massage to help constipation

Abdominal massage makes a huge difference to constipation and there are various ways of doing it.

- Using a belly ball available from www.detoxspecialist.com.au, roll the ball around your abdomen. Start using your right hand on the right side of your body massage up towards your ribs and then across to the other side under your ribs, then down the left side to your groin. You can swap hands or use either hand. It is best to keep the ball under your bed and do this morning and night.

- In the shower, massage with your fingers under your ribs starting on your right side and moving to your left side. If you also alternate the water from hot to cold it will increase the blood flow to your bowel.

- Take both hands and with your palms spread, slap your abdomen 50 times.

- Measure 10mls of olive oil and to this you can add a total of 5 drops of essential oil. To relax the bowel and for inflammation add 3 drops of lavender and 2 drops of German chamomile. To stimulate the bowel add 2 drops of peppermint and 3 drops of rosemary. To help nausea add 1 drop of orange, 2 drops of ginger and 2 drops of peppermint oil. Massage around the abdomen from right to left.

Note: Peppermint and rosemary are contraindicated in epilepsy, high blood pressure and pregnancy.

Tip: Breathing deeply and slowly whilst you massage increases the positive effects.

Cold pack

A physiotherapist told me about this tip for constipation. Get a cold pack (sold in pharmacies) and put it in the freezer. In the morning wedge it on your left side against your psoas muscle which is your groin area near the top of your leg. Use your trousers to hold it up. You can keep it there whilst you drive the kids to school or yourself to work or whilst having breakfast. After 15 minutes to ½ an hour remove it and you will have an urge to do a poo.

Heat

Being warm helps relax the bowel muscles; having a sauna, warm bath or using heat packs on the tummy and back can help bowel movements through relaxation and circulation.

Sit-ups or half sit-ups

A couple of hours after your supper do about 5 minutes of sit-ups or half sit-ups. You can put your feet under your bed if you like, to support yourself. If you have a sore neck put a towel around your neck for support. Hold onto it as you sit up. I have found that for many people this has increased pancreatic function and really helped upper digestion, making a big difference to bloating after meals.

Do a spinal twist

Spinal twists allow excess toxins in the digestive system to be released and have a calming effect. While in a cross legged sitting position, slowly turn to the right and hold while taking a few deep breaths then repeat this process on the left side. You can also bend one leg on the floor and put the other leg over it with your knee up. Do a spinal twist pushing your elbow over the risen right knee. Swap sides and push your right elbow over your left knee.

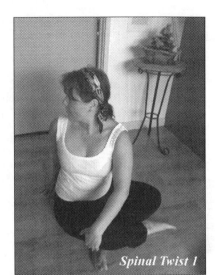

Spinal Twist 1

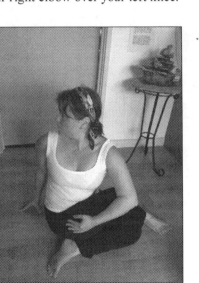

Spinal Twist 2

Massage your valves

Often the valves on either side of your bowel can get irritated (ileocecal and houston valves) or stay open or closed when they shouldn't. To help them, lie on the floor with your knees and lower legs over a bed or chair. Interlock your fingers on both hands over your tummy button. Open your thumbs as far as they go and push them into your abdomen. Your thumbs will be half way between your hip bone and tummy button. Push the tip of your thumb deeply down into your flesh and in the same movement up towards your face. Breathe in and then out as you insert your thumbs. Repeat this 15 times each day and you will really notice the difference. It also benefits you if you have pain in these areas.

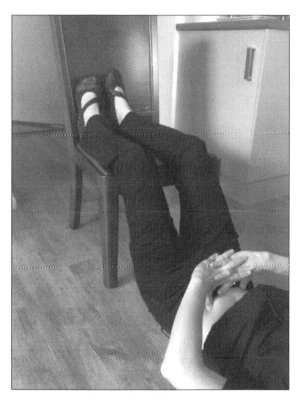

Ileocecal Valve Massage

Belly breathing

Kneel down sitting on your calves. Place your hands face down on or near your knees. Breathe in and out through your mouth, squeezing your tummy in as you do it. You tummy will automatically relax between breaths. Do this repeatedly for a couple of minutes; short sharp breaths, pulling the tummy in with each breath and letting the tummy go in between breaths.

Lymphaciser

Bouncing on one is a great natural laxative, it also strengthens your colon muscles and nerves as well as helping digestion.

Squatting

This makes a big difference to many bowel conditions especially constipation and haemorrhoids.

The way we sit on toilets is an unnatural position for the bowel to evacuate and creates tension on the nerves, muscles and ligaments of the lower colon. Toilet design has not changed for many years and the designers have not taken into account how physiology works otherwise toilets would work for proper elimination. Squatting is a natural position that opens up the rectal canal more easily and allows faeces to pass as gravity does most of the work. Squatting devices are available from are available from www.detoxspecialist.com.au in Australia.

They stop haemorrhoids getting worse and prevent them from occurring as it avoids straining during evacuation.

Going to the loo becomes much more of a relaxing experience.

Squatting also helps the pelvic floor and bladder.

You don't have to wait until you have a problem or injury you can use it as a preventative.

Whilst you are waiting for your squatting device you can start squatting by using two telephone books on either side of the toilet. Lift both the toilet seats up, stand on the books and you'll experience a much easier bowel movement. It also helps keep you more supple. I'm amazed at how easy is it for a lot of Asian elderly to squat because they have been using those muscles all their lives whereas in the west most elderly people can't bend to squat.

Dr. B.A. Sikirov carried out a study, "Management of Haemorrhoids." It showed that squatting for passing stools was both preventative and curative for haemorrhoids.

His study details cases of 20 haemorrhoid sufferers aged between 22 years and 70 years, some with a 20 year history of haemorrhoids. For them, conventional treatments hadn't worked. The study required that each person adopt a squatting posture for passing stools in response to a strong urge.

Sikirov describes the kink in the bowel as primary constipation. The kink is open when squatting.

Crohn's disease

Squatting has also been proven to help crohn's because when you squat it closes off the ileocecal valve preventing bacteria like e.coli entering the small intestine. This valve needs to be supported by the thighs to stop pressure from evacuation.

Appendicitis can be prevented as in a sitting position the caecum cannot effectively empty. This is near the appendix and it can then cause inflammation from stagnation.

The small intestine can be contaminated when bacteria backtrack through the ileocecal valve between the small intestine and colon as mentioned above. It generally stops the backflow of wastes but if the valve stays open when it shouldn't then problems of inflammation in the small intestine can arise. Squatting seals the ileocecal valve which stops contamination or leaking. See massage exercise for the ileocecal valve.

Diverticulitis also benefits from squatting as it can develop from over straining and a blocked colon. Interestingly diverticula have not been found in any wild animals, which says something about our diet and lifestyle.

In severe cases of constipation a 7 day juice fast with enemas or colonics, taking laxative teas and Epsom salt (on the first day) maybe beneficial. For some people a juice fast is inappropriate and they are better with animal stock broths and vegetable soups.

Also consider seeing therapists like osteopaths, chiropractors and physiotherapists as back problems can lead to digestive problems.

CHAPTER 7

How balancing acid and alkaline can help your gut heal

"Beauty isn't something on the outside. It's your insides that count! You gotta eat green stuff to make sure you're pretty on the insides."

Takayuki Ikkaku

Chapter 7
How balancing acid and alkaline can help your gut heal

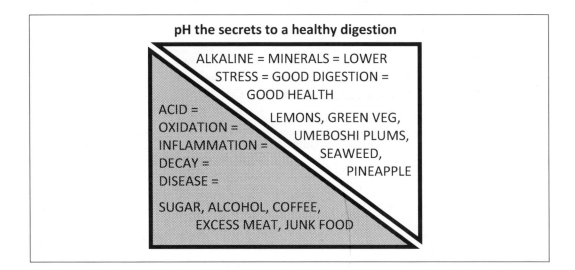

pH the secrets to a healthy digestion

ALKALINE = MINERALS = LOWER STRESS = GOOD DIGESTION = GOOD HEALTH

LEMONS, GREEN VEG, UMEBOSHI PLUMS, SEAWEED, PINEAPPLE

ACID = OXIDATION = INFLAMMATION = DECAY = DISEASE =

SUGAR, ALCOHOL, COFFEE, EXCESS MEAT, JUNK FOOD

Balancing acid and alkaline to help your gut

Over 100 years ago, the American biochemist McQuenn wrote, "The Acid Death of the White Race." This made over acidity the subject of medical research. Professor Schade at the University of Dresden, Germany proved in 1910 that acid accumulation triggers pain. Then another scientist, Ragner Berg from Sweden, developed a theory of acid-base balance in the body that is affected by diet. He relied on the work of Salkowski, who published results in the 1870s that suggested inorganic acids could only be excreted by the kidneys if they were neutralised by inorganic bases. If the acids remained in the body, they would accumulate in areas of low blood flow (like joints), obstructing normal function. The model disease was gout, but Berg traced many other "diseases of civilisation" to acid-base imbalance, including obesity, arthritis and diabetes.

Because the body produces more acids than bases (opposite of acid), Berg concluded, the best source of bases was the diet. If the diet is too acidic, then the body breaks down necessary minerals in the muscles and bones to compensate. Normal chemical processes in the body produce acids and as long as there are the necessary alkaline minerals to buffer the acids, adverse effects aren't experienced.

The intestinal environment has an influence upon the stress of acid within you. If you have a high protein diet there is a shift in intestinal micro-organisms and a shift in pH explained shortly. The waste products of faecal bacteria can then no longer be converted to ammonia and excreted in the faeces. They are absorbed by the body and the liver has to work hard to detoxify them.

Your intestines absorb minerals from food and the acid/alkaline balance is a way of measuring what your absorption and mineral level is like. However, it is not easy for people to balance it effectively today, with fast foods, white flour, sugar, lollies, soft drinks and caffeine which all contribute to acidity.

There are many important tests that health practitioners can do to monitor your health. One test you can do at home yourself is to test your pH (potential hydrogen). This will help you kick-start your diet to healthier choices and give you a reality check. It is tested using a yellow paper or pH strip. You can keep these in your bathroom and 2 hours or more after a meal take a small bit of the paper or a pH strip and urinate on it. It will then change colour and you will have a chart with your kit, so you can see how acid or alkaline you are. Usually more yellow on the chart is acid and green is alkaline. You can also spit on the paper or strip and test your saliva. The saliva pH shows how strong the pancreas and liver are at digesting and the urine pH how acid or alkaline the body is regarding mineral loss. Testing is usually measured on a scale of 1-14. Anything below 7 is acid and above 7 is alkaline. A healthy pH is about 6.2-6.9 which is slightly acidic. If your urine is below 6 this is extreme acidity and you must do something about it or you have every chance of getting a chronic illness if you haven't already. An American scientist, Carey Reams, proved that a pH that is overly alkaline is also a problem and causes a breeding ground for parasites and other nasties.

Reams developed (Reams Biological Theory of Ionization) which provides comprehensive digestive testing, including testing to show how acid or alkaline the body is through saliva and urine. For a deeper more comprehensive look at your digestion, see a practitioner who does R.B.T.I testing (available from www.detoxspecialist.com.au). Your pH is a good start but R.B.T.I. will give you a lot of valuable information about your digestion including your pH. You can buy pH paper from health shops, though I'd also highly recommend R.B.T.I. testing to see the whole picture.

Your blood needs to be constantly alkaline at a narrow pH range of 7.35-7.45 for you to stay healthy and to keep you alive. Your body will take minerals such as calcium, magnesium, potassium and sodium from your muscles and bones in order to keep the blood alkaline if you are acidic. So if your urine is often acidic you are losing precious minerals from your body in order to keep your blood pH stable.

Your urine pH is directly related to both tissue oxygen levels and soft tissue levels of the minerals calcium, magnesium, potassium and sodium. These minerals are vitally important for every cell in the body. If your urine is showing acid then the body is eliminating acid residue and is losing vital minerals. As well as certain foods, fatigue, infection and depletion contribute towards acidity.

Acidic body= inflammation= oxidation=more acidity= decay=disease

One thing that may be confusing for you is that you may have been told to take supplements to increase hydrochloric acid (HCl) in your stomach. This is the only place in your body that you want to have acid. HCl is very important to help you digest your food well and it is one of your first lines of defence. If you eat a lettuce leaf with a parasite egg on it and you have good levels of HCl it will kill it off right there in your stomach and you'll have no further problems, whereas if you have weak HCl, that little egg may make it into your intestines and grow and multiply and cause all sorts of havoc. It is also more likely to grow if your intestine has a low amount of good bacteria/flora.

If your pH is less than 6.2 consider more alkaline foods in your diet and avoid acidic foods.

Alkaline foods include green vegetables, carrots, beetroot, lemons, limes, Celtic salt, pineapple and umeboshi plums (these are Japanese salted plums available from the health food shop).

Acidic foods include sugar, table salt, processed foods, coffee, excess meat, white flour, excess dairy, alcohol, soft drinks, poor quality oils that are heated and anything artificial. These are the main ones but most foods in the absence of vegetables or lemons can make your body acidic.

Water that you drink often has chlorine, fluoride, metals and microbes that can be acidic to the body so it's worth investing in a filter.

The people from the islands of Okinawa, in Japan, are known for their long and healthy lives. They get a lot of minerals from their water and natural healthy food and have a healthy lifestyle. As a consequence they have less than half the colon cancers that Americans do.

Healthy sports drinks and potassium

Ideally potassium should be present inside your cells at a concentration of 30-40 times higher than outside. Potassium is very important and you lose it when you sweat. That's why leading sports drinks contain potassium and without it your heart can stop! Magnesium deficiency can cause this too, however, most of those drinks have nasty artificial additives in them and you are better off drinking coconut water or adding some Celtic salt to your water; about half a teaspoon to a litre. The other thing potassium is important for is taking nutrients into the cells and toxins out of the cells otherwise the toxins get stuck and you may experience not feeling quite right or get headaches.

Emotions that are positive like love and joy help create a more alkaline environment and negative emotions like hate and jealousy help create a more acidic environment. Minerals are also lost from your body when there is physical and mental stress in your life. The Shaolin monks of China and other spiritual leaders are more alkaline because they manage stress with meditation which has a direct chemical effect on their bodies.

Allergic reactions are also a form of stress and produce acids in the body.

Balancing diet

People vary as we all have different lifestyles and makeup but as a general rule having 70% alkalising foods and 30% acidic foods is ideal. When you are on a cleansing diet you may want to eliminate acidic foods altogether. The combination of foods that you eat, how well your digestive organs are working and your reserve of minerals can also affect the outcome of whether a meal is acidic or alkalising. Interestingly with eggs, the yolk is alkaline and the white is acid, probably because it protects the yolk. Still eat the whole egg though and add some spinach leaves or other greens to balance the meal and have an alkalising effect.

Why lemons?

Many people ask how lemons which are highly acidic outside of the body can be alkaline inside the body. Well, they contain citric acid which is a "weak" acid, meaning once it's done its job in providing energy in metabolism it's eliminated easily via sweat and respiration. The acid easily dissolves and alkalising minerals are left which neutralise body acids. It is alkaline forming because it stimulates the formation of calcium carbonate in the body. Calcium carbonate (a buffer solution) then neutralises the "strong" acids in the body, acids that can only be got rid of through urination, including uric acid which is the end result of protein metabolism.

In fruits like lemons and limes the mineral content is also taken into consideration, and lemon is high in buffering alkaline minerals like calcium, magnesium, and potassium, so after the citric acid has done its job and is easily eliminated, you are left with a very alkaline ash (end product) from the fruit. These buffering minerals (sodium is also alkalising but not in refined salt) help sponge the corrosive effects of acids in the body and interestingly, acidic foods like oranges don't have strong alkalising effects because of the sugars (acid) which offset the high level of minerals. In fact, lemons are not alkaline but they have an alkalising effect on the body.

Tip:

Be careful of your teeth as lemons are acid in your mouth but when they reach your small intestine they become alkaline. All you have to do is swish your mouth with fresh water after consuming lemon and spit it out. This will protect your tooth enamel.

Acid foods like flour, sugar, meat and fish leave sulphuric and phosphoric acids behind after being metabolised however, they are not always acidic (except sugar which is a no no). If they are combined well with alkalising foods and the body chemistry is optimal then it can eliminate acid residue. It really is individual for example, if you have colitis that means there has been acidity, inflammation and low mineral content in your body for some time so you will need to up the ante on your alkalising foods and be much stricter with acidic foods. It's the same with most chronic diseases.

Some foods are neutral and they will make the acid less acid by their mineral content and the alkaline foods less alkaline by their protein content for example, eggs and dairy. The main thing is to make sure you get lots of mineral rich vegetables. If you go out and have a coffee and cake you will become acidic but if you eat healthy vegetables later on, you will most likely bounce back however, if you have been acidic or low in minerals for some time you may not bounce back to a healthy pH and that coffee and cake can put you in a negative balance for days. It becomes worse if you have fungus (like candida) or parasites that love sugar. They will multiply from the yummy sugar, produce more acids and toxic by-products which will make you tired and run down.

If you struggle psychologically with taking things out of your diet or you are the type that binges after feeling deprived, then allow yourself that something nice once a week. You are not a rubbish bin; treat yourself like a precious object, you deserve healthy vibrant fresh foods from nature. Most of us are conditioned from childhood that we deserve a cake if we are good which is back to front as it's bad for us. Why not deserve vegetable sticks and healthy dips, vegetables juice, nuts and seeds. Once you get to a really healthy state the odd cake and biscuit will have little negative effect on you especially if you deal well with stress. However, I don't recommend these things as people build up bad habits and often choose sweet foods that are full of artificial stuff. I have a friend who is Greek and as a child she was given red capsicum, celery and carrot sticks with homemade hummus dip when she was down or sick. She remembers being wrapped up in a quilt in front of the T.V. and served these foods. So what does she do now when she's down? She eats these foods as she wasn't programmed to use sweets as a reward.

There can be some confusion about what is acidic and what is alkalising. Some of this confusion has come because potassium raises alkalinity by displacing acidic hydrogen ions (a charged atom or molecule) in the cells. The misunderstanding comes because the acidic hydrogen ions push out of the cells and into the extra-cellular fluid. We cannot measure the higher alkaline pH levels inside the cells, but only the rising acid outside in the extra cellular fluid, saliva and urine so it is said that some whole grains like brown rice (high in magnesium and beneficial) are acidic whereas it's the harmful acid that leaves the cells. Once outside the cells, provided the diet is healthy, the body can buffer the acid and get rid of it through the kidneys.

Minerals and pH

I'd advise you not to get too obsessed with taking your pH and keep your focus on what is right with you whilst improving your health. Once or twice a week is a good way to keep a check of what is happening on the inside. Each 0.1 increase in your pH means a 10 fold increase in tissue oxygen which is a good thing. So if you have an acidic pH of 5 and shift to 7 you'd have a 150 fold increase in tissue oxygen and your digestion will be operating a whole lot better.

An overly acidic pH (and overly alkaline) is a sign of low minerals. Minerals are the most essential substances for the body. They are like the foundations of a house and everything builds on them for example, vitamins cannot absorb properly without minerals. There's no point taking loads of vitamin supplements if you test acid as your absorption of them will be poor.

Minerals will help:

Treat an existing illness.

Prevent an illness from becoming worse.

Prevent vague symptoms from developing into a full blown disease.

Maintain good health and prevent disease.

Minerals are abundant in vegetables (in particular, green leafy vegetables and sea vegetables like seaweed) and vegetable juices.

Many digestive problems come from acidity and poor amounts of minerals in the diet, which leads to poor absorption and elimination and over time makes things worse.

Role of minerals

The role of minerals is vitally important for health and a lack of them contributes to every disease. Pollution, poor soil quality, stress and acidic diets are some reasons why so many people have a lack of minerals.

- They help build teeth, bones, connective tissue and cell membranes.

- All bodily processes depend on the action minerals.

- They help pH as enzymes transform minerals into an alkalising detoxifying agent which combines with acid waste and toxic settlements within the body, neutralising them and preparing them for elimination.

Calcium is the most abundant mineral in the body (makes up 1.5-2.2kg of your body weight) and the efficiency of each mineral is enhanced by balanced amounts of the others. Interestingly, a shortage of just one mineral can disrupt bodily activity rendering other nutrients useless. You lose a massive amount of minerals through your urine, bile (from the liver/gall bladder), sweat and faeces (poo) as a result of normal daily processes in the body. The daily losses usually amount to more than 700mg which must be replaced on a daily basis and what makes you lose more minerals? Sugar, caffeine, alcohol, cigarettes and junk food!

Be careful with calcium supplements; you really need a hair analysis to determine the right calcium for you. Some supplements can lower your stomach acid which isn't good and others can displace calcium into your arteries however, if you need them and take the correct supplement for you, you'll get fantastic results.

The effects of food on your body

If you have poor liver and pancreatic function then this will lead to your food being poorly broken down, poor absorption and poor bowel movement. At the same time, if you are eating poorly farmed foods, processed foods, chemicals, irradiated food and foods that have had a long transportation time more minerals will be lost. A 4 year study in the U.S shows a decrease in minerals on farms with standard agricultural practices. This includes a decrease of 41% calcium, 22% magnesium and 28% potassium. In contrast, other studies show a much higher mineral content in organic fruit and vegetables.

How to stop destroying minerals in your body

- Eat until you are comfortable rather than overeating.

- Eat slowly and chew well.

- Sit for 10 minutes after eating and sit down to eat.

- Avoid toxins like cigarettes, coffee and tea (especially around meals).

- Avoid refined food like sugar and white flour.

- Avoid chemicals in your food and water.

- Some drugs can affect mineral balance.

- Avoid eating when you are stressed.

- Foods higher in potassium, calcium and magnesium (vegetables, seaweed) have an alkalising effect.

- Foods higher in protein and phosphorus (meat) have an acidic effect and eating vegetables with protein helps offset this effect.

Your intestine and acidity

Your intestine is directly involved with acid or alkaline intake from your food and due to different intestinal absorption rates of proteins and minerals in individuals, this can have an impact on pH as well as acidic food intake.

The East is more alkaline than the West

Interestingly, populations around the world with the lowest calcium dietary intake also have the lowest rates of osteoporosis. People in countries like Sri Lanka, Peru, Africa and China maintain healthy bones on 200-500mgs of dietary calcium a day and many western populations have brittle bones on 1500mgs of dietary calcium a day.

Why is this?

In the West, diets have become acidic (too much meat, sugar and junk food) which uses up calcium and other alkalising minerals pulling them from bones and tissue. If you eat more vegetables and have reserves of minerals you can buffer acids from moderate meat consumption. If, for example, you have a 50mg increase in urinary calcium loss by having and acidic diet, this means over 20 years you can lose half of your skeletal calcium! Your gut and nervous system would not be happy and get very tight and tense. You will also exhaust your kidneys as they have to work hard to excrete acids. Studies show that those of you who consume more fruits and vegetables have a higher bone density which means more beneficial minerals for your gut function and other mechanisms in your body. Magnesium is also lost when you are acidic which causes problems with the bowel muscle leading to constipation.

Beware, coke is 100,000 times more acidic than blood, causing a massive amount of work for your pancreas to help buffer the acidity and you lose a lot of your precious minerals to help neutralise the acid.

5 alkalising secrets

1. Start the day with ½ a **lemon** in hot water.

2. Reduce **soft drink.** There are 11tsp. of sugar in a can (sugar free versions are also acidic).

3. Reduce **sugar** or eliminate it. (Use stevia or another natural sweetener instead).

4. Eat more **umeboshi plums;** they are salted Asian plums sold in health food shops. One a day helps the body alkalise.

5. Increase **vibrant greens including seaweed.**

According to Reams, the vegetables celery, parsley, green beans and zucchini are top of the list for the alkalising mineral potassium. You can make a soup called 'Bielers broth' from these vegetables.

If you take out poor quality foods from your diet and increase organic whole foods your need for drugs and supplements will be less. To get a big mineral boost in your diet, incorporate seaweeds like nori and dulse in your diet which are readily available from health shops. They are the highest plant source of minerals and have many health benefits including assisting in healthy thyroid function. Cereal grasses like wheat grass and barley grass are also high in minerals. You can also incorporate sprouts (like mung beans and alfalfa) and vegetable juices for their quality, taste and vital force.

If you have a tendency to any digestive problem including a virus, parasite, fungus or mucus problem you need to manage stress, have a more alkalising diet, exercise and drink healthy water. You will find healthy herbs and alkalising recipes (not the desserts) in Ch.11 and 12, in particular the salads and drinks.

Over the last century the western diet has become more acidic robbing the body of minerals. Life has also become more stressful with less exercise for many of you. An alkaline, moderate protein diet can greatly benefit your digestive and overall health and reduce disease.

CHAPTER 8

How to choose good and bad oils

"Keeping your body healthy is an expression of gratitude to the whole cosmos - the trees, the clouds, everything."

Thich Nhat Hanh

CHAPTER 8
How to choose good and bad oils

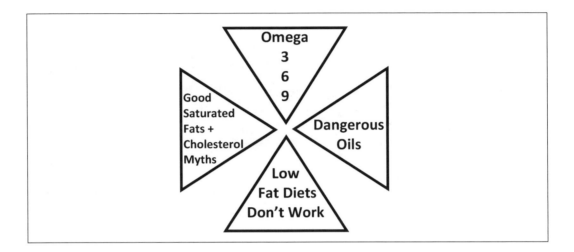

Fatty acid facts

Growing new research has found concerns in our understanding of fat and why fat is important in nutrition. Good fat is very important for the lining of the intestine. Commonly, fat is associated with the heart which is a relatively new disease and now kills 1 in 3 adults.

It has been linked to obesity which alarmingly kills 2 out of 3 Americans. Medical experts have said this is due to over-eating fat but it's the carbohydrates that actually do it. Obesity puts pressure on all the digestive organs, stomach, bowel, pancreas and liver as well as the heart.

It is very important to understand what fats are good for you and your digestion and what fats are bad. Drugs for lowering lipids (blood fats) and cholesterol are the largest selling drugs with sales reaching over 24 billion dollars. These drugs have side effects and in some people too much fat and cholesterol is being taken out of the body, affecting digestion and memory.

Fats we eat

The fats we eat are made up of a variety of fatty acids each containing a chain of carbon atoms with two hydrogen atoms attached to each carbon.

Saturated

Now when all the carbon bonds that are available are occupied by a hydrogen atom the fatty acid is called saturated. These fats are very positive to the body and as they are so stable they can withstand high temperatures. The atoms are squashed together tightly which means the fat is solid or thick. Most saturated fats come from animals or tropical plants like coconut oil and palm oil. They are important for taking fat soluble toxins out of the body.

Unsaturated

I'll just use a little more basic chemistry to explain the difference with liquid oils. When a hydrogen atom is missing in the carbon chain the fatty acid is unsaturated.

These oils are unstable and do not withstand high temperatures.

Why?

Well, what happens is that a double bond is formed when two carbon atoms, even lacking one of their hydrogen partners, join together. There are destructive things called free radicals (unpaired electrons) that destroy your cells and these bonds attract free radicals making unsaturated fat prone to damage. Double bonds form a bend in the chain and so they don't pack together so well and they stay liquid rather than solid.

Polyunsaturated

Later I will talk about omega 3 oils as they are polyunsaturated fats. These are very unstable and should not be heated but kept in the fridge. As you will see however, they are essential for the health of your body which includes the cells of your digestive system. They are great for inflammation in the digestive system.

Monounsaturated fats

They have only one double bond so they are more stable than polyunsaturated fats but not as stable as saturated fats. They can be heated but it's not advisable as you have to keep the temperature very low. Oleic acid is the most common monounsaturated fat and is found in almonds, avocados, olive oil, and pecans.

So how did confusion arise?

In 1957 a nutritionist, Ancel Keys, researched heart disease and diet across six countries. His research stated that coronary artery disease was related to saturated fat. Some time later he realised that if he had four times the number of countries in his research his conclusions were no longer valid. He attempted to dispute his original research but was ignored and the food industry was on its way to making big changes. Gone was healthy animal fat and lard and in its place came unsaturated fat which is not stable and was used more in packet food and cooking.

Unfortunately, Aneel's original findings were backed by cardiologists and the cholesterol, arteriosclerosis and heart disease theory around fat was founded on faulty research. This has led to digestive problems from cutting out fat and over consuming carbohydrates and sugar.

Low fat diets

Fat doesn't make you fat. It's the low fat diets that cause you to crave carbohydrates which raise insulin which makes you fat. The first recorded case of heart disease was in 1910 but before that, people ate 300% more saturated fat including lard and other animal fat and they didn't have the digestive and other health problems we have today.

Then the fad started with low fat diets and did they work? No! People craved food and ate more carbohydrates and became unwell from fat deficiencies. Fat is necessary for the uptake of fat soluble vitamins A, E, D, K and carotenoids. Polyunsaturated fats are essential for reducing inflammation, particularly in the gut and are necessary for managing colitis and crohn's disease.

We are supposed to eat whole foods as nature intended, not take the fat out of milk or other products, because fat is necessary for the uptake of the above vitamins. When it is taken out of milk, calcium is poorly absorbed and calcitrol, which is the hormonal form of vitamin D, is suppressed. Vitamin D is vital for bone health and preventing cancer but it also has a host of other benefits.

Absorbing fat in the gut affects fertility and ovaries

In a U.K. fertility study involving 18,000 women with fertility problems, because of a lack of egg release, two or more servings of low fat milk was responsible for an 85% increase in infertility. They summarised that full fat milk contained a fat soluble substance that improves ovarian function. This substance makes milk more absorbable in the gut. Butter also helps. I'd only recommend organic milk and even better, raw milk where they use clean practices to milk the cows. You can get it by buying shares in a cow! The fat removed from milk contains "Wulzen factor," and it is this that protects you from arthritis. If calves are fed skimmed milk they develop joint stiffness and do not thrive.

Interestingly, in the famous nurses study involving more than 80,000 people, one or more serves of low fat milk was linked to a 32% higher risk of ovarian cancer.

Conjugated linoleic acid is found in full fat milk and is anti-cancer and immune boosting (most of the immune system is in the gut) but it is lost in low fat milk.

Saturated fat is actually good for you!

There are several researchers who have shown that saturated fat is beneficial for you, including Weston Price. If you look at "The Weston Price Foundation" there are so many beneficial tips on diet. He found that people living in Northern India consume 17 times more animal fat but have 7 times less coronary heart disease than people in Southern India.

Even more interesting is the famous Framington Heart Study which began in 1948 and involves 6000 people. They set out to prove that saturated fat was bad but the director was forced to admit "We found that the people who ate the most saturated fat and cholesterol had the lowest levels of serum cholesterol, weighed the least and were the most active." So does that make you feel better? You can go out and eat saturated fat from animals, though I recommend grass fed or organic as toxins collect in fat and remember to have vegetables with these proteins to keep the body more alkaline. Fat is very healing to the gut and helps to remove toxins that are attracted to the fat from your body, for example, some heavy metals and pesticides.

How does saturated fat work in your body?

Most of your nutrients are absorbed through your small intestine which is just below your stomach. These nutrients do many things including providing energy for the heart to pump blood around your body and to keep the blood healthy and strong. The fat around the heart is highly saturated as this is the preferred heart food in times of stress. About 50% of dietary fat needs to be saturated and it helps good calcium absorption for your bones. A diet rich in saturated fats helps essential fatty acids (mentioned later) remain in the tissues of the body.

When you have more of these fats you will get fewer colds and flu as these fats boost your immunity and have been shown to lower bad cholesterol (LDL).

Many people have nasty microbes and parasites in their gut and saturated fats, which include short and medium chain fatty acids, protect against these nasties. What's more they also protect the liver from alcohol damage and drugs however, that doesn't give you permission to get drunk or high on drugs! But if you are a recovering alcoholic or detoxing from the silly season, these fats are very useful. Fats are to be taken in moderation; more than 30% in the diet can be difficult to digest and saturated fat in excess contributes to constipation.

Digestive health is worse for carbohydrates

Fat has more calories than carbohydrates but if you don't have fat you will crave carbohydrates as fat makes you feel full.

Carbohydrate is stored as fat if you eat too much of it. Your pancreas produces insulin in response to a rise in blood sugar from carbohydrates and if this is continually repeated eventually your pancreas will burn out and you are at risk of diabetes. You have a higher risk of diabetes if you are obese. I urge you to think seriously about this as when I was a nurse, a lot of diabetic patients had legs amputated because they went black with gangrene and they also became blind as a result of diabetes. They often expressed words to the effect, "if only I'd realised this might happen I would have looked after myself more." Insulin removes excess glucose from the blood (a sugar in carbohydrates) and stores it as something called glycogen and then as fat. The more insulin you produce the more fat you get as insulin blocks the release of the fat-burning substance, glucagon.

Is cholesterol really bad?

Cholesterol is really important to strengthen the cell membranes of the bowel wall and is very useful for leaky gut. It is also necessary to produce certain vitamins which in turn help the gut.

Cholesterol is also very important for hormone production which, in turn, has an effect on the gut. It is also vital for brain health and high cholesterol diets have has been shown to be beneficial for people with Parkinson's and Alzheimer's.

Another advantage of cholesterol is that it boosts your immune system and is an antioxidant. It is only a problem if it oxidises and your naturopath can test for that.

Why is it that people with normal cholesterol sometimes have a heart attack? Cholesterol testing is not a good indication of heart health; instead testing homocysteine, C-reactive protein and fasting blood glucose levels will give a more accurate picture. More than 60% of heart attacks occur in people with normal cholesterol and in 20% of cases there is low cholesterol! When arteries are becoming blocked, cholesterol comes in to make them more pliable and soften the blockage.

This may shock you: A study at Yale University found that old people with high cholesterol had half the number of heart attacks than others their age who had low cholesterol. In another study, doctors from London's Imperial College found that high cholesterol was protective during heart failure. Interestingly, survival "increased by 25% for every mmol/l" of cholesterol.

To help the oxidation, eating antioxidant rich foods helps e.g. blueberries, blackberries, raspberries, acai berry, goji berries and greens like dunaliella salina, chlorella, wheat grass and barley grass. As mentioned earlier, homocysteine and C-reactive protein tests are far better for an accurate measure of heart health. These can be done along with bowel tests through your health practitioner. High cholesterol can also indicate heavy metals and thyroid problems.

Often the main reason cholesterol can rise is when the liver is not efficient at detoxifying or producing enough bile. The liver makes cholesterol and eating globe artichokes helps manage it in a healthy way. The liver is an important part of efficient digestion. Eating more green leafy vegetables and including lemons in the diet also helps the liver. Cholesterol rises to protect the body from an onslaught of toxins. Rather than killing cholesterol with drugs (that have their own side effects, including neurological and memory problems, lymphatic cancers and heart issues!) why not think about the message they are giving and addressing the cause of the problem.

The other thing to be aware of if you are on statins is that they lower an important nutrient called co-enzyme Q10 which is essential for heart function.

Safe and unsafe oils

What I will mention before I discuss Omega 3 oils is that the only oils that are safe to cook with are: coconut oil and rice bran oil and animal fats like butter, ghee and lard, because they are stable under high heat. Cold pressed sesame oil is a polyunsaturated oil resistant to rancidity as it contains a natural preservative called sesamol. It needs to be used at very low temperatures and is best added at the end of cooking for flavour. It contains high amounts of vitamin E and 43% omega 6, calcium and lecithin which are good for the brain. It is also good in salads. Research has shown that sesame oil contains a lignin sesamin which lowers blood pressure over a 60 day period. It is also helpful in diabetes.

Avocado oil has the highest smoke point out of any plant oil but still needs to be used at a low heat. It is used as a flavour enhancer and is best added to salads an hour before serving. It is also great in Asian dishes. Research shows that 1½ tablespoons of avocado oil added to a salad increased the carotene uptake by 720%, beta carotene by 15% and lutein by 510%. So it is worth adding to food to boost the uptake of nutrients to help immunity which is especially useful for crohn's, colitis and inflammatory bowel disease. It is also a penetrating skin food and an amazing moisturiser.

Other oils change their molecular structure under high heat and are very harmful to the body. Unfortunately these oils are used in most takeaway foods. Most cheap vegetable oils have been solvent extracted which destroys valuable antioxidants. These include soybean, sunflower, corn and cottonseed oils; I'd advise you to avoid these.

Fats that have had hydrogen put into them to make a polyunsaturated oil solid like margarine (hydrogenated) are also harmful to the body. These are known as trans-fats and are toxic to humans. Margarine is naturally grey and bleach, dyes and flavours are used in it to mimic butter! It's sold as a healthier alternative but let me assure you, butter is much better for your health and is a rich source of vitamin A. Just put a small plate of margarine and a small plate of butter outside and watch as the insects crawl over butter and nothing living will touch margarine! It's only one molecule away from plastic! For 50 years we thought margarine was healthy and now we know it can be deadly.

Look out for hydrogenated oil, or partially hydrogenated oil in packet food. This is used as a preservative and cheap fat like margarine and is not good for you. Commercially, some margarines have had plant sterols added to lower cholesterol and this is an awful assault on your health. Yes it works but you then have all the side effects of the margarine. Trans-fats are so unhealthy the digestive system doesn't recognise them as they are not natural and they go into your cell membranes. This wreaks havoc with cell metabolism. Consumption of hydrogenated fats has been linked to many diseases including: digestive cancers, atherosclerosis, diabetes, obesity, poor sight, low immunity, sterility, birth defects, bone and tendon problems.

Avoid these and protect your children and family from all the processed foods that contain them. They need to be removed from catering, processed food, tuck shops and take-aways. They are in a shocking 40% of supermarket foods including: margarine, biscuits, peanut butter, soups, dips, snacks, ice-cream and salad dressings.

I will mention again, these hydrogenated fats are **really bad** for the digestion.

Avoid canola oil. Although it is very popular, it has its issues. Modern canola was hybridised to shut down heart damaging erucic acid but new studies are showing that even the small amounts that remain may still cause heart lesions. Canola goes rancid easily and during the shelf extending deodorisation process, the 12% omega 3 content in canola is transformed into trans-fats. It is not suitable for cooking as it oxidises easily.

All oils are better if they are organic and cold pressed.

Lack of Fat

As I've mentioned, over the years people have avoided fat because they thought eating fat would make them fat. People who avoided fat often got dry skin, skin diseases, cancers and other problems. Now people have more awareness on the benefits of eating fat. Omega 6 and omega 3 fatty acids are required by the body in equal amounts but because of the saturated fat phobia many consume a vast amount of omega 6, which in excess stops the absorption of omega 3 and omega 3 is less likely to be consumed. Whilst a balance is needed, too much omega 6 can lead to inflammation and a constriction of your arteries.

People generally lack short chain fatty acids found in butter and cream. These fats defend against digestive parasites and are rapidly absorbed for instant energy.

Omega oils

So getting to Omega 3; there are 3 types of omega oils - 3, 6 and 9, all beneficial to your health in the correct balance. A healthy diet should consist of roughly 2-4 times fewer omega 6 fatty acids than omega 3 fatty acids as explained in the table below. The typical Australian diet, however, tends to contain 14-25 times more omega-6 fatty acids than omega 3 fatty acids. Many researchers believe this is a significant factor for the rising rate of inflammatory disorders.

Omega Oil	Description
Omega 3 (EPA and DHA)	There are 2 main types of omega 3 fatty acids. The second is mentioned in the next column.
	1. Long-chain omega 3 fatty acids are known as EPA (eicosapentaenoic acid) and DHA (docosahexaenoic acid). These are abundant in fatty fish.
	Omega 3 fatty acids are essential nutrients for health. We need omega 3 fatty acids for numerous normal body functions, such as:
	controlling blood clotting,
	lowering high blood pressure,
	inhibiting cancer tumours and building cell membranes in the brain, and since our bodies cannot make omega 3 fats, we must get them through food. Omega 3 fatty acids are also associated with many health benefits including:
	helping <u>inflammatory bowel disease, and other autoimmune diseases such as crohn's disease</u>.
	helping depression,
	other mental illness,
	improving brain function,
	healthy skin,
	protection against heart disease
	and possibly strokes.

Omega Oil	Description
Omega 3 (ALA)	2. Short-chain omega 3 fatty acids. These are a source of polyunsaturated fatty acids ALA (alpha-linolenic acid) and are found in plants such as flaxseed.
	They are used to treat the same conditions as long-chain omega 3 fatty acids.
	Though beneficial, ALA omega 3 fatty acids generally have less potent health benefits than EPA and DHA. It is hard for the body to fully convert ALA to EPA and DHA so that omega 3 is effectively absorbed. You have to eat more to get the benefits you do from fish oils and your body has to have vitamins such as B3, B6, C and co-factors magnesium and zinc to absorb it well and convert it effectively. These oils decrease inflammation and are useful for rheumatoid arthritis and all the other inflammatory bowel diseases mentioned above.
	Both Omega 3s can have a marked effect in helping weight loss due to inflammation in the fat cells that a lot of overweight people have.
Omega 6	Omega 6 fatty acids are also polyunsaturated, such as linoleic acid (LA).
	Linoleic acid is converted to gamma-linolenic acid (GLA) in the body. It is then further broken down to arachidonic acid (AA). GLA is found in several plant oils. Omega 6 fatty acids lower LDL cholesterol (the "bad" cholesterol) and reduce inflammation, and they are protective against heart disease.
	They play a crucial role in brain function, as well as normal growth and development, they help stimulate skin and hair growth, maintain bone health, regulate metabolism and maintain the reproductive system.
	So both omega 6 and omega 3 fatty acids are healthy. Omega 6 is useful in breast inflammation, ADHD, osteoporosis, diabetic neuropathy, PMS, menopausal symptoms, rheumatoid arthritis, eczema and multiple sclerosis.
	As mentioned, a lot of people have too much omega 6 and an absence of omega 3.

Omega Oil	Description
Omega 9	Omega 9 is the most abundant fatty acid in nature and is not in short supply in our diets. Omega 9 fatty acid is a monounsaturated fat that is also known as oleic acid.
	Omega 9 is not technically an <u>essential fatty acid</u> because the body can produce a small amount, provided the essential fatty acids omega 3 and omega 6 are present.
	If the body is low on one of these EFAs it cannot produce enough omega 9. In this instance, omega 9 transforms into an essential fatty acid because of the body's inability to produce it.
	It plays a much smaller role than omega 3 and omega 6.
	Primarily, omega 9 has a positive health effect on the lowering of cholesterol levels and it promotes healthy inflammation responses within the body. Other major health benefits of omega 9 include the reduction of insulin resistance, improvement of immune function and it provides protection against certain types of cancer.
	Omega 9 supplementation is mainly used when there is an insufficiency of either omega 3 or 6 or both.
	Omega 9 fatty acid foods
	Mustard seeds
	Peanut oil
	Safflower oil
	Virgin olive oil
	Olives
	Avocado
	Nuts and nut butters
	Pecan
	Pistachio
	Cashew
	Hazelnut
	Macadamia
	Almond

A note on supplements and food:

Long-chain omega 3 includes fish or a good fish oil which will contain about 400mg of EPA and 200mg of DHA. However, for specific needs it is best to contact your naturopath, as ratios alter for different ailments. The fish oil will turn yellow if it's rancid (off). It is important that they are transported/kept in a refrigerator.

Coconut oil is fantastic for cooking and using in your diet to help weight loss, for blood sugar balance, immunity and candida but it doesn't have omega 3, so you need to mix your oils to get different nutrients.

Short-chain omega 3 fatty acids - vegetarian options include **flaxseed/oil, chia seeds** and hemp seed/oil.

Flaxseed oil comes from the seeds of the flax plant which in latin is usitatissimum meaning "most useful" and the fibres are used to make textiles. The ground seed is better than the oil in the respect that it is enriched with the antioxidants, vitamins and minerals needed. It is best to grind it yourself and keep it in the fridge to prevent rancidity. If flaxseed oil is off, it will taste rancid. Flaxseed oil is best bought with added vitamin E as an antioxidant to protect it and sold in a container that allows no light into it. It must be kept and transported in a fridge.

Dr. Johanna Budwig was a German biochemist who specialised in fats and oils in the 1950s. She claimed that a diet high in flaxseed oil and organic cottage cheese could prevent and cure cancer and many other diseases.

In her European cancer research she found that cancer patients are deficient in certain lipoproteins that were needed to counter the harmful effects of hydrogenated oils and trans-fats.

The combination of cottage cheese and flaxseed oil apparently delivers the necessary lipoproteins.

Budwig has thousands of grateful survivors who validate her theory.

The Budwig recipe

1 cup of cottage cheese

2½ tablespoons flaxseed oil

2 tablespoons freshly ground flaxseed

Enough water to make it soft

Optional - a dash of cayenne, honey and fresh fruit. Blend all ingredients.

Other Budwig recommendations: No sugar, no margarine, no hydrogenated oils, regular freshly squeezed vegetable juices, sauerkraut and two tablespoons of freshly ground flaxseed with yogurt every morning.

Her protocol has achieved amazing results with bowel cancer, stomach ulcers, bronchial spasms, enlarged prostate, arthritis, eczema and multiple sclerosis.

Chia seeds are a wonderful source of omega 3 and can easily be added to your diet. Originally from South America, they are now grown in Australia. Chia is an ancient seed that has more omega 3 and dietary fibre than any other natural food.

Until recently it hasn't been grown here and was not part of the Australian diet as it requires specific climatic conditions to grow. It is now being grown in the Kimberley region of Western Australia, exactly 15 degrees from the equator to produce the best quality chia.

Chia seeds contain omega 3 ALA. It can be sprinkled onto any food and is great in porridge. It becomes jelly-like when wet and is easy to assimilate. Chia can also be added to smoothies. You can buy black or white chia seeds and they are nutritionally the same.

A tablespoon provides all your daily requirements of omega 3 ALA. It is a really good source of fibre (great if you suffer constipation) and protein. Like flaxseed they need to be converted.

Chia seeds are also good for weight loss and increasing satiety – so you will feel full for longer. They also help steady blood sugar. With a unique combination of soluble and insoluble fibre, they will keep your energy stable rather than a series of ups and downs during the day. Chia oil is now available and must be refrigerated. By weight, chia contains more omega 3 than salmon and it still tastes like whatever you want! It's also recently been targeted as a weight-loss helper however, it's not as easy to convert as salmon oil.

USA weekend magazine reports on a study where overweight dieters who included omega 3s in their eating plan lost two more pounds monthly than the control group, who did not. This is most likely because inflammation in the body was reduced by the oil.

Hemp seed oil is more balanced than flaxseed oil. Flaxseed oil is very rich in omega 3 but by using it exclusively for too long in the absence of other omega 6 oils you may develop cracked, flaky skin after 10 months. Hemp oil can be used long term as it contains a healthy balance of omega 3 (20%) and 6 (60%) and gamma linoleic acid (2%). It tastes like sunflower oil and is green. This oil also contains an amazing 35% soluble fibre. Hemp seed and flaxseed oil need to be refrigerated and never cooked with. Flaxseed can be balanced by omega 6 rich oils like sunflower and sesame.

UDO's oil is another good choice for vegans and vegetarians and it contains a healthy blend of omega 3, 6 and 9 in a balanced ratio. Dr. Udo Erasmus is a leading expert in oils and has a bestselling book for further reading, Fats that heal – Fats that kill and Choosing the right fats.

Other healthy oils

Macadamia oil is produced in high amounts in Australia. It has 5 times more vitamin E than olive oil and a higher smoke point but best used uncooked or at very low temperatures.

A study in the Newcastle research project revealed significant reductions in inflammation and clotting tendency associated with consuming macadamia oil. It also increases good cholesterol (HDL) and is beneficial for inflammatory bowel problems and stomach ulcers.

Apricot kernel oil is cold pressed from the seeds of the apricot. It is great for salad dressings, has a nutty flavour and a high level of vitamin A and E for healing, which is useful for the bowel lining. It is nutritious and used a lot in skin care.

Rice bran oil (such as King rice bran oil) is good for cooking as it has a high smoke point (213°C), it has a mild flavour and is a thin oil to cook with which some people prefer compared to coconut oil. A component of the oil oryzanol was shown in Japan to be effective in relieving hot flushes and other symptoms of menopause. Researchers found 90% of the women found some form of relief from hot flushes after taking rice bran oil for four to six weeks.

The antioxidants including vitamin E in rice bran oil are not destroyed at high temperatures. It is not easy to get this oil organically.

Coconut oil - Last but not least, coconut oil has a huge number of benefits. Dr. Mary Enig is also an expert on fats especially coconut oil and her leading book about coconut oil and weight loss is, Eat fat lose fat. It has been shown to help with many health related problems including thyroid, candida, digestive disorders (it kills pathogens associated with diarrhoea), parasites, weight loss, melanoma, diabetes and energy increase.

Coconut oil is a saturated fat but unlike other saturated fats has medium chain fatty acids which don't stress the pancreas or liver and they are not stored as fat but sent directly to the liver where they are converted to energy. This fat keeps you full but doesn't put on weight. You can add a tablespoon to your porridge, cook with it, mix it with plain yogurt, use it as butter, add a tablespoon to hot water or drink it for energy.

Coconut oil contains lauric acid which boosts the immune system. Lauric acid is part of breast milk and protects against pathogens.

When coconut oil became cheap in the U.S. pig farmers used it to fatten their pigs but instead of fattening them they became more lean!

Cooking with unsaturated oils can cause cross-linking of molecules, fragmentation and all kinds of molecular damage that is much worse than trans-fats. Coconut oil withstands high heat and gives you health benefits however, you still need other oils for other benefits like omega 3 and vitamin E.

In 1978, Sri Lankans consumed an average of 120 coconuts each per year and yet heart disease was only 1 in 100,000. This has changed, since the introduction of cheap, damaged polyunsaturated oils which has affected these people.

Coconut oil is beneficial in diabetes as it helps stop sugar cravings and provides nourishment to the cells. With a lack of insulin in diabetes, cells starve as insulin tales glucose and fatty acids into the cell. Arteries weaken and nerves become damaged. Amputation, blindness and kidney failure are unfortunately all common outcomes. The medium-chain fatty acids in coconut oil are small enough to enter the cells without insulin so they offer some nourishment in type 1 and type 2 diabetes. Coconut oil also increases the production of insulin so is a must in a diabetic diet.

Animal studies have shown polyunsaturated fats consumed in excess cause cancer. In one study every animal developed tumours except those fed coconut oil. Those fed coconut oil were also immune to chemically induced breast cancer and to induced skin cancer if the oil was applied topically.

Polynesians coat their bodies in coconut oil and don't suffer from skin cancer. We need a variety of good oils including omega 3, 6 and 9 so it's all about balance.

The beneficial dose of coconut oil is 1-3 tablespoons a day according to your needs and toleration of fats.

How you choose oils in your diet is very important for digestive and overall health. Eat oils that come straight from nature, pure, organic and unadulterated and only cook with oils that are not damaged by heating them.

Avoid fats used in take-away food but include good fats in your diet as they only have a positive effect on the body and stop you overeating by satisfying your hunger.

For specific health advice, always contact your naturopath or health care professional.

CHAPTER 9

The art of fermenting for digestive health

"Make your own recovery the first priority in your life."

Robin Norwood

CHAPTER 9
The art of fermenting for digestive health

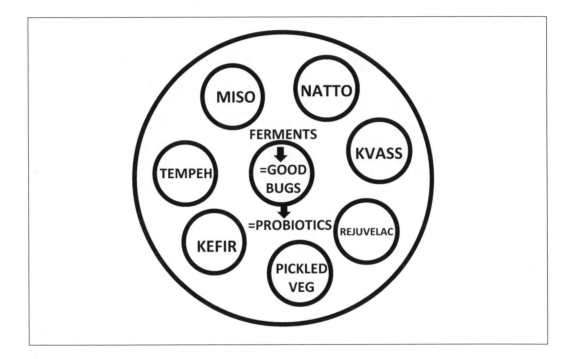

Bowel Miracle

Probiotics/Flora - What are they and how do they work?

Believe it or not there are ferments that aren't alcohol and they have a very positive effect on your health. Fermented foods are the oldest form of helping healthy gut flora dating back some 5000 years.

They are a wonderful health food as they help gut ecology and encourage hundreds of species of micro-organisms in the gut (bowel). For centuries, fermented foods have been used in many cultures throughout the world and it is one of the oldest preservation methods. It is even more prevalent in rural communities and making fermented food is cheap and easy.

Fermented foods and drinks have adapted over time and vary in different regions. For many cultures it is an efficient, low cost preservation method that decreases the need for refrigeration and unnatural modern preservatives.

There are a huge number of good organisms in your gut, in fact they outnumber the number of cells in the human body, or at least they should if you have a healthy gut. You have over 9 metres or 30 feet of digestive tract from your mouth to your anus and 100 trillion good organisms living there. These weigh 2 kg which is even heavier than the weight of your liver! When you have good bugs there is a massive 40% difference in mineral uptake from your diet.

These micro-organisms not only help digestion but also absorption and the immune system in the gut. As about 70% of your immune system is in your gut it is very important to keep it healthy.

The good micro-organisms (flora) prevent the bad bacteria, nasty parasites and fungus from overtaking the gut and playing havoc with your health. These good micro-organisms can play a significant part in the recovery of irritable bowel, inflammatory bowel, bloating, poor digestion and crohn's disease to name a few.

Your gut is assaulted on a daily basis. Just look around the supermarket at the abundance of processed food that can sit on shelves for weeks without spoiling. You put that into your gut and the same thing happens, it stops spoiling and affects good flora. The natural bacteria aren't allowed to break it down effectively as it's been tainted with preservatives to stop it breaking down. It doesn't stop there; you may also drink water containing chlorine. Why is this bad? The chlorine kills off your healthy bacteria. Get a filter, even a cheap one to start with. Prescription drugs like the pill, stress and alcohol all affect your flora. We have an epidemic of digestive problems and zantac (for digestive problems) is one of the biggest selling drugs.

Flora in your gut can have different purposes. Some flora helps more when taking antibiotics, other flora maintains bowel health. Specific flora helps eczema, allergies and immune support and yet other flora helps yeast infections, traveller's diarrhoea and gut inflammation. Although the gut contains hundreds of species of good flora there are two main species which you may have heard about, these are: *Lactobacillus acidophilus or acidophilus* and *bifidobacterium or bifidus.*

Acidophilus is found more in the small intestine whereas *bifidus* is found more in the large intestine.

Bifidus is the most important flora for babies and represents 99% of the beneficial bugs for them. It is very protective of the immune system and helps produce B vitamins.

When you take antibiotics it can take 6 months of having probiotic supplements to get back to the same state of good gut organisms you had before. However, because probiotics are not eaten from a live fermented culture they do not necessarily keep replicating in the gut, so you have to keep taking them to replenish your bowel, as they can die off in the gut after a few weeks of stopping them.

Healthy fermented foods are in a culture and help lay good flora down in your gut. There are many countries that eat 3-8 forms of fermented foods daily. During fermentation there is a slow breakdown of organic substances by micro-organisms or enzymes from food. Oxidation (a chemical reaction of a substance exposed to oxygen like an apple turning brown) of carbohydrates occurs changing the biochemistry of the food and when salt is added it prevents the food going off, which can happen from toxins being produced by organisms.

Why are fermented foods so good?

In some situations the balance of the flora in the gut is so bad that you may find you are constantly sick with tummy troubles and immune problems yet you often don't know that you are lacking bowel flora. Fermented foods may not have a high enough count of certain organisms for specific conditions but long-term they can make a significant difference to gut health. If you do take probiotics get the advice of a knowledgeable health practitioner so you get what is best for you.

Fermentation neutralises anti-nutrient chemicals found in grains for example, phytic acid (anti nutrient is something that uses up more nutrients than the food has or takes nutrients out of your body) which is in some grains and particularly high in oats, can block the absorption of calcium, iron and zinc.

Fermentation creates a host of beneficial micro-organisms in food increasing its digestibility. When food is fermented it breaks down the cell wall and makes the absorption of the nutrients in the food better. It can also increase the nutritional content of the food.

You may never have eaten fermented foods before or understood why you need to eat them. Some of the foods I'm about to mention, you may not have even heard of but just open yourself up to the possibility of eating some and then enjoy making some yourself. It's actually an exciting creative journey. As you experiment you will experience the wonderful health benefits of these foods which can make a significant improvement to your digestive and overall health. For example, kefir, which I will talk more about later, has helped so many people. If you look on the internet people have even written songs about this amazing drink!

Who are fermented foods for?

Fermented foods and beneficial organisms will make a significant difference to:

- Anyone wanting to improve their gut and general health.

- Preventing problems as we age, as digestive enzymes do diminish with age.

- Those who have had or are on antibiotics.

- Allergies.

- Skin complaints like eczema, psoriasis and acne.

- Irritable bowel.

- Fungal infections like thrush and candida.

- Gut inflammation and bowel disease.

- Bacteria in the stomach like Helicobacter Pylori.

- Bad breath.

- Those who are on or who have taken medication that disturbs gut flora in particular the pill and steroids.

- If you have had gastro or have picked up a parasite at home or overseas.

- To protect your health when travelling.

- To increase immunity especially those for that have conditions where immunity is suppressed and the more fragile members of society, those sick and convalescing young children and the elderly. Most autoimmune problems start in the gut so it is beneficial for all autoimmune conditions and to prevent them.

Advantages of traditionally fermented and pickled foods

- They encourage the growth of beneficial micro-organisms in the gut like *L. Bacillus* and *L. Bulgaricus* which promote intestinal health.

- Flavours are improved or intensified e.g. soya sauce, miso, kim chi.

- Beneficial enzymes develop and this makes food easier to digest, especially proteins, and it improves the uptake of nutrients.

- Certain nutrients increase e.g. vitamin C in cabbage, protein in tempeh and B vitamins in cultured milks.

- The food is preserved which increases the shelf life and decreases the activity of the micro-organisms involved in food spoilage.

There are many types of fermented foods made from vegetables, cheeses, fruits, grains, dairy and soy.

Let's have a look at how to make some of these:

Fermented foods and how to make them

Fermented foods may seem totally foreign and a bit overwhelming to make. Start with one recipe that appeals to you and master that before going to the next. The good thing is none of them need cooking!

REJUVELAC

Rejuvelac is a non-alcoholic fermented liquid made from sprouted grains. Rejuvelac can be drunk as a digestive aid or used as a starter culture for other ferments.

Properties and benefits

It aids digestion and contains 8 of the B group vitamins (important for energy and helping stress reduction). It also contains vitamins E and K, and a variety of proteins and carbohydrates. As with other fermented foods it is packed with probiotics.

Cooked grains take a lot of energy for the pancreas to digest and the rest of the digestive system to break down; by sprouting grains, your body finds it easy to digest and it enhances your digestive function and makes it easy to break down. If you don't ferment grains, soak the grains overnight before you cook them to remove phytic acid and make them more digestible.

Ingredients

2 cups of your choice of organic wheat, rye, quinoa, oats, barley, rice, millet or buckwheat grains. Unhulled grains are better and need thorough rinsing.

Filtered or spring water.

Instructions

Place the grain of your choice in a glass jar and fill it ¾ full with water.

Soak for 8-12 hours and then rinse the grains.

Rinse the grains 2-3 times a day until you can see tiny white tails appearing.

Rinse the grains well and place in a 2-3 litre glass jar.

Fill the jar with spring or filtered water and place a tea towel or cheesecloth over the jar and then place a rubber band over the jar to hold it in place.

After 48 hours it is ready. Drain the rejuvelac and store it in the fridge.

Place the sprouted grains back in the jar and fill ¾ full with spring or filtered water.

The second batch will be ready in about 24 hours.

Pour rejuvelac through a strainer and put it in the fridge. Then discard the grains into the compost.

Tips: Rejuvelac should appear yellowish, cloudy and tart, slightly carbonated and not too sour to taste.

Every batch can be slightly different. Some batches are stronger and some weaker.

Sometimes a fine, white mouldy-looking layer forms on the top. Just scrape it off. It is harmless but always use your nose to determine if it is good to drink or not.

BEETROOT KVASS

Properties and benefits

A small glass of beet kvass morning and night is great as a blood tonic, digestive regulator, helps remove acid from your blood, liver cleanser and overall healing tonic. What's wonderful about it is that it keeps things moving! You need to get used to the taste as it's not like alcohol or soft drink. Once you've had it a few times you will enjoy the buzz it gives you.

Ingredients:

3 medium or 2 large beetroots peeled and chopped coarsely
¼ cup whey
1 tbsp. salt
Filtered water

Method:

Place beetroot, whey and salt in a 2 litre glass container. Add filtered water to fill the container. Stir and cover securely. Keep it at room temperature for another 2 days. The first brew that you make will be less strong than the second brew. After the second brew is made, discard the beets and start again. You can reserve some of the liquid and use this as your starter inoculation instead of whey.

Tips: Avoid grated beetroot as it exudes too much juice resulting in rapid fermentation that favours the production of alcohol instead of lactic acid. If you are going out, avoid purple hands by wearing rubber gloves when peeling beets. They actually make a great natural dye and you can colour children's food with beetroot juice.

PICKLED BEETROOT

Ingredients:

12 medium beetroots
Seeds from 2 cardamom pods
1 tbsp. celtic salt
4 tbsp. whey (if not available add another tbsp. salt)
1 cup filtered water

Method

Prick the beetroots in several places, place on a baking sheet and bake in a low oven for 3-6 hours or until soft. Peel and cut into ¼ inch pieces. Place beetroot in a glass container with a wide mouth and press down with a meat hammer. Combine the remaining ingredients and pour them over the beetroot. Add more water if necessary to cover the beetroot. It is best if the tops of the beetroots are at least 1 inch below the top of the jar. Cover tightly with a lid or cloth and keep at room temperature for 3 days before putting it in the fridge.

Tips: Avoid grated beetroot as it exudes too much juice resulting in rapid fermentation that favours the production of alcohol instead of lactic acid. You can also use turnips and onions. Beetroot is a good source of iron.

Pickling with salt and apple cider vinegar

You can buy a vegetable press from a health food shop and add shredded/grated vegetables and a couple of teaspoons of salt. The lid has a press and within 24 hours the cellulose membrane of the vegetable will break down and water will emerge. You can put the fermented vegetables in a glass jar and store it in the fridge; they last about a week.

Alternatively, you can put the vegetables and salt in a bowl and add another bowl (take care with glazes as they can leach heavy metals; use white glazes) on top with a heavy weight in it and this will act as a press. Leave this for 24 hours then store the vegetables. Pressed vegetables not only aid your digestion, they are so easy to digest because the process pre-digests them. Vegetables like cabbage, carrots, broccoli, cucumber, greens, and daikon radish are suitable.

Apple cider vinegar can have spices added to it like cloves and ginger. You can add a small amount when pressing your vegetables as above. The vinegar enhances the digestive process in the stomach.

Tips: Aside from fermenting you can add a tablespoon of apple cider vinegar to 50mls of water and sip this with your meals to enhance digestion. Whilst other vinegars are harmful for candida and fungal infections, apple cider vinegar actually helps these conditions. Outside the body it is acid but inside the body, like lemons, it is alkaline. The pancreas produces a buffer solution that helps it alkalise your body. You can add it to salads with olive oil and garlic.

SPICY KIM CHI

Ingredients:

1 green or red cabbage chopped

1 green or red cabbage juiced

4 large carrots chopped

4 large carrots juiced

¼ cup freshly grated ginger

1 tbsp. cumin seed

1 tsp. dried red pepper, ground

1 tsp. miso

¼ tsp. turmeric powder

¼ tsp. cayenne pepper

3 cloves garlic chopped

Method:

Blend carrot juice, cumin, cayenne, red pepper and miso. Mix all ingredients with a spoon and place in a jar, making sure vegetables are covered with juice. Cover the jar by placing several cabbage leaves on top. Put a weight on top of the cabbage leaves and allow it to ferment for three or four days.

Tips: This is delicious on its own and also as a side dish to help your meal digest well. Sterilize the spoon and jar beforehand.

Soy foods

Fermented soy foods include miso, tempeh, some soy sauces and natto. You can buy these already made up from a health food shop.

Non fermented soy foods like tofu, soybeans and soy milk do not have the same health benefits as traditionally fermented soy foods. Soy milk in particular can be mucus forming, difficult to digest and detrimental to health. Many of these foods are heavily processed.

MISO

It is a salty very nutritious paste that can be used as a soup and is used as a breakfast cereal in Japan. It is made by fermenting soybeans or soybeans with rice and barley with a starter called koji.

Koji is made by inoculating steamed rice with the fungus Aspergillus Oryzae. The rice or barley koji is added to the soybeans and allowed to ferment in wooden casks. The colour and flavour of miso depends on the ingredients and length of time it is left to ferment or age; between 6 months and 2 years. See recipes for a delicious miso soup.

Properties and benefits

It is high in protein and highly bioavailable as the enzymes in the koji starter break down the protein. It is very high in B vitamins which are essential for your nervous system. It is a very easy to digest, nutritious food for those who have a weak digestion or want something quick and easy. I wouldn't recommend it for those with candida as fungus sometimes feeds off it.

Tips: Unpasteurised miso contains live cultures and abundant lactic acid forming bacteria. Miso reduces and eliminates radioactive substances from the body so it is great for those exposed to x-rays, electromagnetic radiation and environmental radiation. It is rich in substances called isoflavones, genestein and daidzin. These are thought to be invaluable in cancer, especially stomach cancer. These substances are created in the fermentation process.

Storage

Store miso in the fridge. Shiro is the sweetest miso and hatcho the strongest. They are generally made from soybeans and husked grains of roasted brown rice and will last several years. They are best kept in glass (transfer from the plastic container you bought it in) never boil it but add it at end of cooking to preserve nutrients and enzymes.

Add a teaspoon to a cup of hot water (with a bit of cold water) and tear up some nori seaweed for a quick nutritious soup. (see Ch.11 for details on seaweed) You can also spread it on a rice cake as a paste and add avocado on the top.

TEMPEH

Tempeh is originally from Indonesia. It is made from whole soybeans fermented with a grain such as rice or millet. The starter culture is Rhizopus Oligosporus which forms a mould that causes a mat like web to link the beans together. It is fermented for 24 hours to form a chewy cake. The fibre content is high because whole bean is used.

Properties and benefits

Tempeh is a very good source of iron, magnesium, zinc and B6. It is common if you have gut problems to be lacking in nutrients and iron will be lacking anywhere there has been a small or large bleed. It goes well with beetroot which is also high in iron.

It is very high in protein and comparable to beef or chicken and it is easily digested for the compromised gut. It also has lots of fibre which again is easily absorbed and non-irritating for the gut. Tempeh has minerals and omega 3 oils due to the fermentation process. It also contains the substances genestein and daidzin which have anticancer and antioxidant properties.

Fermentation increases the bioavailability of nutrients from the soybeans. Consumption does encourage the growth of bacteria which produce B12 in the intestine however, there is controversy regarding its effectiveness.

It has long been assumed that B12 is produced by bacteria in the large intestine (the colon/bowel), but since B12 is produced below the ileum (the lower end of the small intestine, where B12 is absorbed), it is not available for absorption. This theory is reinforced by the fact that many species of totally or primarily vegetarian animals eat their faeces! Eating faeces allows them to obtain B12 on their diets of plant foods.

Herbert reports on this theory in a study in the 1950s in England where vegan volunteers with B12 deficiency (as shown by megaloblastic anaemia) were fed B12 extractions made from their own stools (yuck!) and it cured their deficiency.

He said it proves that the bacteria in the colon of vegans produces enough B12 to cure a deficiency, but that the B12 produced by the bacteria in the colon is excreted rather than absorbed. This appears to be convincing evidence. I certainly wouldn't recommend you do this but if you are vegan or vegetarian get your B12 checked every 6 months as symptoms of deficiency can be horrible and affect memory, the spinal cord and nerves. If you are deficient, a supplement is a bit easier than eating your own poo, or consider changing your diet so you get B12 in it!

As well as helping digestion, fermented soy foods have been the subject of many promising studies showing that they help the prevention of osteoporosis and menopausal symptoms.

Storage

When you buy tempeh it will look dry on the outside with grains tightly bound like mushroom. Don't be alarmed if there is a white coating, it is normal. You can freeze tempeh for up to a year or keep it for up to 25 days in the fridge.

How to use it

It can be marinated, grilled or fried. The secret to tasty tempeh is in the cooking. It needs to be sliced very thinly and tastes best if a little coconut or rice bran oil is added. Cook each side until it is brown. I cook it with turmeric, garlic and onions. For tasty recipes see Chapter 12.

TAMARI

Is traditionally fermented soy sauce without added wheat. So this is good for celiacs and those with a wheat or gluten intolerance.

SHOYU

Is a similar tasting sauce made by mixing soybeans with grain (usually wheat) and then adding moulds allowing the mixture to ferment in a salty brine for 12-18 months. Microbial enzymes split the proteins into amino acids, producing a salty sauce. Cheaper soy sauce is made by chemical hydrolysis and is not beneficial for your health.

These are healthy seasonings, unlike sauces that have lots of additives and are not natural. You can add them at the end of cooking, or to salad dressings and in dips. They are high in salt so you need to keep your fluid intake up and be aware if you are on a low salt diet.

It is not recommended for those with candida or fungal infections as it can feed the fungus in some cases.

NATTO

Is made from barley, barley malt, soybeans, kombu, ginseng and sea salt. It is a delicious sweet condiment used widely in Japan.

Properties and benefits

It is used like a pickle or chutney. It has an enzyme in it called pyrazine which gives the distinctive odour of smelly feet! I can assure you it tastes a lot nicer than it smells; sweet and nutty. This is a wonderful super food for the gut and great for anti-ageing. It contains another enzyme Nattokinase which has an anti-coagulant (thins blood) effect (in the sticky coating). It has been a staple food in Japan for 1000 years. Natto is very easy to digest and great for those with weak digestion.

Natto has been used with success in place of Warfarin in people with vascular problems in the retina (causing blood clots to form in the retina) in Japan.

It may have a role in preventing osteoporosis as it contains a form of vitamin K (K2) which is involved in bone formation along with calcium. The calcium is very well absorbed due to the polyglutamic acid found in the sticky part of natto. Generally, people with osteoporosis have low levels of K2 and those without have high levels of K2. Osteoporosis can be a problem with chronic malabsorption and celiac disease.

Antibiotic effect

If you have any type of bowel infection this is a wonderful food to add into your diet to help. Natto was used as a medicine before antibiotics for dysentery, typhus and other intestinal diseases. It has even been used to treat and prevent salmonella infection.

KEFIR

Have you tried kefir before? This is another of nature's powerful antibiotics and is made from milk. It doesn't have to be made with cow's milk. You can make it with sheep's, goat's, cow's or even camel's milk if you can find a camel! You can also make it with seed milks like sunflower.

Most people who are intolerant to milk can tolerate kefir as the milk protein is predigested which means it is easily digested and unlikely to cause food sensitivities. Interestingly, those who are lactose intolerant can handle yoghurt because the lactose converts to lactic acid.

It is a soured milk product similar to yoghurt though not as sour as yoghurt. It is balancing and cooling according to Ayurvedic medicine.

It has a smaller curd size, is easier to digest and is more liquid in consistency than yoghurt. It was originally used as a druid brew made from raw goat's or cow's milk. It is cultured from gelatinous particles called grains which contain a combination of bacteria and yeasts.

It is a natural mild laxative which is high in probiotics (good flora) and far higher than yoghurt! It is such a wonderful super-food and has helped thousands of people with gut problems.

Properties and benefits

There are some extra beneficial strains of natural bowel flora not found in yoghurt e.g. lactobacilli caucasus, acetobacter and some streptococcus species. It also has L. caseii, bulgaricus and acidophillus. As well as that, it contains the beneficial yeasts, saccharomyces kefir and torula kefir that disable pathogenic yeasts in the body. It is such a great food for stimulating healthy micro flora in your bowel wall. Kefir also contains bacterial inhibitory factors preventing the growth of pathogenic bacteria that cause stomach bugs. It even protects against bacteria like salmonella and e. coli, which cause severe diarrhoea.

The World Health Organization has reported that kefir has been used to effectively lower typhoid fever and tuberculosis. As many people with gut problems are anxious it is beneficial as it alleviates anxiety due to high tryptophan levels (which converts serotonin in the brain resulting in a relaxing effect).

Nutritionally, kefir is a complete protein, it is high in B vitamins and the uptake of nutrients (especially B12 and B1) is greater than other foods because of the fermentation.

Immune effects

Kefir increases immune function which is necessary for bowel infections, parasites, candida, colitis and crohn's disease. It has been used to help in cases of AIDS, cancer and chronic fatigue.

In cancer, the nonpathogenic organisms in kefir control and reduce the development of carcinogenic substances in the large bowel. High lactic acid in the diet such as in kefir, has been connected to a lower cancer risk.

Kefir is used to help restore balance to your inner ecology which is important for optimal colon health. It can be used for many gut disturbances including diarrhoea, diverticulitis, colitis, constipation, crohn's, dysbiosis, flatulence, colitis, irritable bowel syndrome, systemic candida, gastritis and stomach ulcers. These conditions benefit greatly from including this amazing food in your diet. It also helps with ageing as with age, enzyme systems slow down leading to impaired digestion.

Therefore, fermented foods are excellent for the elderly too. Kefir is also an excellent food post operatively as it helps with bowel function. We find it helps a lot of our colonic clients and after people have had colonoscopies, as this procedure can get rid of a lot of good flora. It has a delicious taste and texture.

You can buy kefir starting grains from health food shops to make it yourself. It is very easy to make, all you do is add the grains to a milk of your choice and leave the mixture in a glass container on the bench and within 24 hours it's ready to eat.

Kefir and yoghurt are delicious as lassis, smoothies or with stewed or poached fruits. It can be used to replace mayonnaise, coleslaw or potato salad or put on rice or buckwheat. It can be used in recipes instead of yoghurt but won't have the same bioavailability when cooked.

You can buy it ready-made but it is best to make it yourself for freshness and an abundance of probiotics.

Be aware when buying cultured milks to look for live or active cultures on the label and avoid those labelled low fat and look out for additives.

Make kefir part of your daily diet. You only need a small shot each day but it's tempting to overdo it with all its wonderful properties.

Storage

In the fridge as you would do with yoghurt.

Staying healthy and combating viruses, bacteria and parasites can be a continual challenge. Ingesting probiotics in fermented foods are an important part of a dietary plan to enhance wellness and combat illness. Probiotics clearly have valuable attributes for your intestines and overall well-being.

CHAPTER 10

Why detoxify and what are the challenges?

"Pain (any pain- emotional, physical, mental) has a message.
The information it has about your life can be remarkably
specific but it usually falls into one of two categories."
We would be more alive if we did more of this" and "Life
would be more lovely if we did less of this" Once we get the
pain's message and follow its advice the pain goes away."

Peter McWilliams

CHAPTER 10
Why detoxify and what are the challenges?

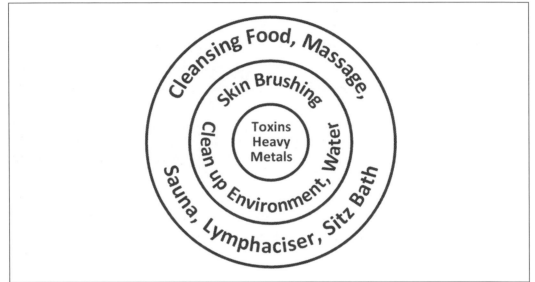

Living the Detox Lifestyle

Detoxification

Keeping your digestion healthy and staying healthy can be a challenge in the modern world. Your body has a natural ability to get rid of harmful substances through your organs which include the liver, kidneys, gastrointestinal tract (stomach and bowel) and the skin. Sometimes the demand on these organs is too much. With modern lifestyles you are exposed to a lot of toxins, for example through food (like additives, preservatives, colouring, processed and junk foods), drink (like alcohol and soft drinks), cigarettes, recreational drugs, medical drugs, environmental pollutants (including car fumes, heavy metals and pesticides) building materials in your home, electromagnetic radiation, cleaning products and make-up.

Your body was not designed to cope with the abundance of toxins that are now part of modern lives. A French scientist Dr. Alexis Carrell kept chicken heart cells alive for more than 27 years through a program that fed the cells nutrients and cleansed cellular waste. They only died when his successor stopped cleansing the cells. This shows that both cleansing and proper nutrition can aid longevity and vitality.

Toxins not only come from your external environment, they can also be generated in your body from stress, unfriendly bacteria in the gut, yeasts and parasites in your digestive system. These internally generated toxins can be absorbed into your bloodstream affecting your health and energy. An important strategy for a long healthy life is regular cleansing and nutrition to fuel your detoxification.

Most of us will be lacking in essential nutrients to aid detoxification and sometimes the body just can't keep up; it gets tired and weary. In 3 generations we have lost 80% of the nutrition in soil and have processed nutrients out of foods.

Sometimes you may push your body with excess work, or overload it with junk food but eventually your body becomes run-down and you can end up with chronic or acute illnesses. Both to prevent and treat illness we can all benefit from a detoxification program.

When you see a qualified health practitioner they will usually do tests on your organs and design a program for you which can include herbs, homeopathy and nutrients. There are many detoxification programs and it can be confusing to know which one to do. I wouldn't advise anyone to go out and buy herbal products; it is best to do that with someone who knows their stuff. What I will give you are simple safe ways you can detox at home with diet and lifestyle techniques to help you feel younger and more alive however, if you have a medical condition get advice from your health practitioner first.

More energy is involved in the process of your body detoxing than any other process in the body and your body has to do this on a daily basis. By giving the digestive system a rest, your body is able to utilise energy more effectively for getting rid of unfriendly toxins. A detox is needed to increase longevity and achieve quality of life.

Is toxicity the reason you feel unwell?

Ask yourself the following questions:

Are you often tired or lethargic?

Do you suffer from bloating, diarrhoea, constipation, nausea, bad breath or farting/gas?

Do you get regular headaches?

Are you suffering from muscular aches and pains?

Does your memory and concentration affect your ability to function well?

Do you suffer from allergies, environmental sensitivities or intolerances?

Do you suffer from depression, anxiety and or mood swings?

Do you have hormonal problems or excess weight?

Do you have skin problems like rashes or pimples?

Do you get swollen glands, runny nose, wheezing or frequent colds?

The more questions you answer yes to the more toxic you are likely to be.

Detoxification is about eliminating toxic substances that cause problems in your body and giving your body a chance to recharge with healthy whole foods and juices.

Ideally, give yourself a minimum of three weeks to cleanse your body and do this at least once a year. Once you have done it for three weeks you will have developed new healthy habits that will stick. If you are healthier, each time you do a detox you will feel better. Ideally you don't want to keep trashing yourself in order to justify a detox; you'll enjoy the benefits from a detox now and then due to modern-day toxins which are all around you.

So the aim is to cleanse using several approaches which include:

Removing the load on your digestive system: avoiding alcohol, cigarettes, drugs (unless they are a necessary medication) sugar and processed foods.

Renewing your body by providing it with essential nutrients: eating fresh organic foods, drinking purified water and vegetable juices.

Releasing toxins through the digestive tract, liver, kidneys and lymphatic system: using simple whole foods and herbal teas to support your organs as they remove wastes.

Replacing and improving the good bugs and renewing your digestive lining: eating foods that help get rid of bad bugs and foods that promote good bugs (Ch.9) and removing waste from your digestive system.

Relaxing is most important for repair and recovery.

Most people are not functioning at their full potential and committing yourself to cleansing is an effective way to give your body a fresh start and get you feeling young and alive. It will allow your cells to renew and change your body to a healthier chemistry. If your body is overwhelmed with toxins and not able to clear them effectively then it loses its ability to maintain a high level of health.

What is a toxin?

A toxin is any substance that can harm your body and is not natural for the body. As mentioned earlier, most toxins come from exposure to environmental pollutants, poor dietary choices, produced from parasites and fungi living inside you and from your own acid wastes.

Some people have good functioning kidneys, liver, skin, lymph and bowels and therefore can get rid of toxins easily but others have reduced function of these organs and these organs can get more sluggish over time if they are overworked or lacking in nutrients. So if you stop putting toxins into your body and help your organs of elimination to get rid of existing toxins effectively, you'll start to see great results.

Giving up cigarettes can cause stress and if you prepare 6 weeks before you start, you can minimise this. Increase vegetable juices, have colonics and stop sugar. Give yourself positive suggestions and practice relaxation: "I feel wonderful now that I have stopped smoking. Every cell in my body benefits and I'm healthy and vibrant."

What are pollutants?

Pollutants are chemicals released into the environment that have a harmful effect on the body e.g. pesticides, herbicides, dry cleaning fluid, hairspray, cosmetics, deodorants, antiperspirants, toothpastes, heavy metals, x-rays, EMR, fly spray, dry cleaning and industrial chemicals. The average woman applies 126 chemicals in 12 products to her hair, face and body everyday! There are many natural alternatives. Diesel exhaust particles settle in the lungs and bladder and studies implicate an increased cancer risk. Heavy metals and pesticides take a long time to break down in the environment and accumulate in the food chain, especially in animal tissue. This is another important reason to eat organic meat, grains, fruits and vegetables not only whilst detoxing but also to stop toxins building up.

Environmental pollutants are so far reaching there is no clean ice on the planet and even the breast milk in Eskimo mothers has been found to contain dioxin which is a hazardous waste.

Plastics contain a toxic substance known as phthalates which are in toys, furniture, storage containers, communication appliances and baby's bottles. Avoid plastic toys or at least only use hard plastics. Most teething rings have 40% of leaching phthalates. The harder the plastic the fewer phthalates, so cling film being soft and flexible is very high in phthalates and is used to cover food. Use baking paper from the health shop to wrap sandwiches and use sealed glass containers in the fridge rather than cling film. Please do not use microwaves, especially for heating food in plastic. Phthalates pile up in the body and your body doesn't get rid of it unless you detox; we're not designed to cope with modern day toxins. Phthalates also leach off gas from plastics on phones, switches, wires and furniture.

If you buy plastic storage containers for food, make sure they are **BPA** free as this is also harmful to your body.

Dioxins are class one carcinogens and damage hormones. They come from industrial smoke and a contaminated food chain. They have been found below 20 feet in the Arctic! Cancer hardly existed in children in 1900 (only from hazardous professions like chimney sweeps), now it's the biggest killer of children and dioxins and other toxins are a major causative factor. Dioxins are in pesticides and block hormones contributing to endometriosis, infertility and loss of libido. Eat organically and start to become aware of how you can avoid environmental pollutants and manage them by detoxing.

Fragrance exposure can be polluting. It is estimated that five million Australians are experiencing harm from synthetic fragrance exposure. Natural essential oils are a better choice for creating nice smells. Other pollutants include industrial smog, exhaust fumes and incinerators. You may think that you are safer inside your home but many homes are 100 times more toxic than the outside air.

Most carpets contain more than 12 toxic chemicals.

Phenols from chipboard, formaldehyde from treated wood, chemicals in foam in bedding, toxins from fly spray, cockroach and ant bombs and the list goes on!

Electromagnetic radiation from smart metres, Wi-Fi, computers and phones.

Start to use your common sense and you will soon realise which substances aren't good for you.

Where possible you can buy natural paint, chemical free furniture, natural building materials and neutralise EMR. with geocleanse. Avoid wet carpet shampooing as it brings up toxins and can contribute to mould.

Heavy metals

They are toxic and have increased with modern living. They include arsenic, lead, mercury, cadmium, nickel, aluminium and tin. Minute amounts of these metals can accumulate in your body tissues causing lots of health problems. Some heavy metals have a synergistic effect, for example, lead makes mercury up to 100 times more toxic. Testing for heavy metals is best done through a hair analysis, as the hair picks up deposits deep in the tissues underneath the skin. InterClinical Laboratories offer the most reliable and comprehensive Hair Mineral Tissue Analysis service, and also provide interpretation of the results by a number of qualified practitioners.

Mercury. The largest source of mercury is from amalgam filings in teeth which converts to methyl mercury and stores itself first in the brain, then the pituitary gland which is the master gland and from here it filters to the adrenals, ovaries and other parts of your body. Mercury storage in the body is made worse with acidity. Common symptoms include depression, M.S. type symptoms and chronic fatigue symptoms. Mercury is highly toxic and the American Dental Association found that dentists with moderate mercury toxicity experienced memory loss, confusion and anxiety.

A group of American dentists attempted to sue their own association. They claim that the association has ignored evidence that fluoride in water and mercury fillings can be harmful to the body. The Swedish government, on the other hand, have taken steps towards banning the use of mercury for fillings. The first ban was for pregnant women because of the risks of mercury to the developing foetus.

Cadmium. This has a strong link to prostate cancer, gut problems, arthritis, depression and ringing in the ears. It is in cigarettes but phosphate fertilisers are the largest source, mainly used for root crops. It takes 1000 years to break down. It is also in incinerated plastics, batteries, ceramics and recycled animal sewerage (some manure). Foods high in zinc help offset cadmium, like pumpkin and sunflower seeds.

Aluminium. It has a strong link to Alzheimer's and is found in baking powder and aluminium pans. It is often in sugar and salt as an anticaking agent, soft drinks in aluminium cans, most deodorants and foods like some tomato paste is produced in aluminium vats.

Lead. The body treats it like calcium and it gets into your bones as calcium is displaced. It tastes very sweet and kids have commonly licked old lead based paint. It can lead to anxiety, learning disabilities, insomnia, deafness, aches and pains. There are no laws in Australia about ceramic dinner sets brought in from countries like China. These can contain lead and cadmium. It is in leaded petrol, lead crystal, batteries, tobacco and some canned food from overseas is soldered with lead. Foods high in vitamin C help, like, berries, lemons, limes, parsley and capsicum.

Pectin in apples, coriander, seaweed, fibre and bentonite clay help take out heavy metals. Glutathione is a useful nutrient and is naturally stimulated by turmeric. Often strong nutrients are needed, as in some cases food isn't enough, and these can be prescribed by your health practitioner.

What are free radicals?

Free radicals are a normal part of oxygen metabolism; we all have them and providing we have enough antioxidants to mop them up there isn't a problem. However, it is unlikely most people have enough, as nowadays there are over 87,000 registered chemicals in widespread use; of which 62,000 can cross cell membranes and harm us and we are marinating in them!. The chemical load can be huge!

Free radicals are highly reactive molecules in the body that can damage your cells and contribute to serious health problems like, bowel disease, arthritis, diabetes and cancer. Exposure to some toxins and normal biochemical processes in your body that aren't supported by enough nutrients can cause free radicals to occur.

Antioxidants are molecules that can get rid of free radicals, preventing damage to your cells. Fresh organic vegetables, fruits and herbs are a high source of antioxidants. Whilst you are detoxifying it is important that you get enough support from your diet to protect your cells.

What happens during detoxification?

During detoxification, toxins are cleared from your body. It is important to support your body with healthy food and water as a lot of toxins sit in the fat cells and lymph underneath your skin. As they mobilise into the blood stream you want them out of your body with minimal impact. This involves neutralising toxins through the liver and helping their removal out of the bowel and via the kidneys, lymph and skin.

When you change your diet, lifestyle and make better choices this reduces the intake of toxins and helps toxins to eliminate through your organs. Most people regularly service their cars and clean the pipes; it's time to treat your body to a service. It can seem overwhelming at first until you plan, organise and decide to start. It's a bit like cleaning out your garage of rubbish that's built up over years and it feels really good to get rid of it.

As your energy increases through detoxing, your motivation to keep up the good habits will increase. If you can't start, just do one small thing to make a difference to your health and commit to it for 100 days. Then start with something else, this time you may find you can do more than one thing and build on it in a way that you can achieve something good for your health. You may cut down from four cups of coffee a day to one or have brown bread instead of white, go back to butter instead of margarine, have fruit for snacks instead of biscuits, walk to work or climb the stairs instead of taking the lift.

Whatever you choose, make it real and achievable for you so you can feel proud of the changes you've made rather than a failure. You might like to plan what you will do over twelve months and then look back and see what you have achieved.

Side effects

Whilst you are detoxing you may experience some uncomfortable feelings of nausea, mild headaches and digestive changes. They are usually just symptoms of withdrawal from substances like caffeine, sugar or getting rid of toxins. These should only be mild and will pass after a couple of days. You may need a lot more water to minimise the effects. If you have any severe symptoms contact your health practitioner but it is unlikely there will be a problem.

Keep focusing on the end result, how good you will feel and how kind you are being to your body. Any side effects will soon pass and the benefits will help you in the long term, so it's worth putting up with niggling problems along the way. Some people feel good all the way through a detox program.

As your body rejuvenates you will feel lighter, more vibrant, your skin will glow, your eyes will be clear and sparkle, ailments will start to go and your friends will comment on how well you look.

You will have the comfort and confidence of knowing exactly what you put into your body and that you've been in control.

Program

We all have different lifestyles, medical histories, constitutions, genetics and types of toxicity and the process for detoxification is individual. Detox in a way that you feel you can cope with. Ideally, do it when you are on holiday or have a break from work and it will be easier and better for you in the warmer weather.

The aim is to:

Cleanse, rebalance, repair and support your gastrointestinal tract (bowel and stomach)

The most important part of your body when detoxifying is your gastrointestinal tract as this is where you digest food, absorb it and eliminate waste food and toxins. You want to support the good bacteria and digestive juices as well as prevent reabsorption of toxins. It is vital that your bowels are eliminating easily and you are not constipated.

When cleansing the body it is important to get the immunity, circulation and elimination strong to allow the passage of toxins out of the body. It is also essential that your cleansing organs are working effectively to eliminate toxins; the kidneys, liver, skin, lymphatics, bowel and circulatory systems.

Liver

The kidneys do a bit of work detoxifying but it's mainly the liver that takes harmful substances out of the body. When the liver is detoxifying it goes through two phases of detoxification known as Phase 1 and 2.

Phase 1 rearranges the toxins into a form that phase 2 can deactivate for removal from the body via the kidney or bowel. For these phases to work well they require specific nutrients. If there aren't enough nutrients for phase 1 it can go too fast and phase 2 then has a back up of toxins to process which can make you sick. Or if phase 2 is lacking in nutrients it can be too slow and the toxins can cause a cascade of harmful effects to your body.

You may be referred for a liver detoxification test to a laboratory like Healthscope.

Intestinal gut permeability also plays a role in detoxification. Increased gut permeability allows for increased absorption of toxins, which are processed and removed by the liver, which puts more demand on liver detoxification. Impaired gastrointestinal integrity can be improved with dietary support including prebiotics, probiotics (Ch.9) and fibre.

The following foods help liver detoxification

The sulphur in garlic and onions, selenium in brazil nuts and garlic, B vitamins in brown rice and quinoa, vitamin A in butter and carrots, C in lemons, and E in nuts and olive oil, calcium in tahini, seaweeds, sardines and yoghurt and protein foods for amino acids.

Antidepressants and other drugs shut down the liver's detoxification system often leading to environmental sensitivities and other health problems. Zantac is a common drug given for digestive problems and it has been shown to increase food allergies even months after discontinuing its use.

Reduce toxins and help your organs to detoxify

The liver plays a big part in your digestion and if you need extra support you may need herbs from your health practitioner. A lot can be done with diet, like using lemons in water, consuming a cup of dandelion root tea and bitter greens. Lifestyle support for other organs includes epsom salt baths, saunas, hot and cold showers, colonics, skin brushing, deep breathing, meditation and gentle exercise like walking, yoga and tai chi.

Restore and revive your body

Good nutrition will help restore your health, repair cells and revive your body.

So how do I start?

First of all, start eating healthier foods so it's not a shock for your body. Open your kitchen cupboards and get rid of processed food, sugar and anything that's not healthy. Start to reduce caffeine or eliminate it to avoid withdrawal symptoms.

Buy some pH paper and test your pH before doing a detox. If your urine pH is below 6.2 then you are too acidic and need to build up minerals with soups, vegetable juices and lemons in water. It is best to test your pH two hours or more after a meal. When you are acidic you are not able to absorb minerals effectively from food and supplements and your body will start taking minerals from your bones and muscles to try to equilibrate your pH. When your pH is 6.2-6.6 you are ready to start.

Making it work

Allow yourself time to organise and plan your food. Minimize your commitments and take time out for yourself. Go to the markets or organic shops and stock up with fresh vegetables, lemons, grains like quinoa, brown rice, millet, buckwheat and amaranth. If you need to, you can freeze foods for the days that you don't have enough time to prepare right away.

Lifestyle Support

It's important to treat your body holistically, relaxing your mind and organising rest in your lifestyle to help the process of detoxification.

Easing stress

Stress has a huge impact on all diseases including bowel disease. Immunity is lowered and precious magnesium and B vitamins are excreted which causes more stress.

Take as much out of your life as possible and avoid situations that make you feel stressed. Take half an hour a day to do something that really relaxes you and feeds your soul. Talk to friends to ease worries. Stress has a big impact on health and it's important to relax for long term recovery and to prevent disease. Aim to reduce your workload and resolve conflicts. You can do a variety of things to help relaxation such as yoga, visualisation, deep breathing, meditation, counselling, personal development, tai chi, qi gong, massage, exercise, bathing in essential oils and magnesium salts, music, reading, art and gardening. Make your home a relaxing place and watch less T.V. especially the news!

Clean up your environment

The most common pollutants you need to get rid of to detoxify your environment are those around your home. Have a look under your sinks and get rid of toxic cleaning products. You can clean effectively with bicarbonate of soda and or vinegar. You can also use special microfibre cloths that require no cleaning product.

Have a look in your bathroom cupboard and remove deodorants with aluminium and chemicals, perfumes, chemical moisturisers, cleansers, harmful first aid products, toxic make up, hair spray, soaps, washing machine detergents and shampoos. Even personal lubricants can be toxic; Sylk is a very good alternative. There are a lot of healthy choices now at health food shops, online and through your health practitioner. You can use essential oils like rose and jasmine for perfumes, organic and natural make-up, natural deodorants or bentonite clay with a couple of drops of essential oil. Coconut oil makes a great cleanser and moisturiser.

Put some Epsom salts or cactus plants around your computer to help EMR. Switch off your wifi.

Avoid solvents, petrochemicals and air your house daily leaving the windows open as much as possible. Have the window open slightly at night so you are breathing fresh air. Fans are wonderful ionisers for the air; invest in ceiling fans or overhead fans. Take electrical equipment out of your bedroom and use organic cotton or bamboo sheets.

If you live in the city, see if you can get to the countryside at weekends for fewer car fumes, and environmental pollutants. There's nothing like nature and fresh air to renew the mind and body.

Avoid recreational drugs

The three most commonly used recreational drugs in the western world are caffeine, tobacco and alcohol. These can have harmful effects, putting a load on your liver and they take valuable nutrients out of your body, making you more susceptible to acidity which leads to disease. Aim to stop them or at least cut back. Green tea is lower in caffeine and is high in antioxidants, so is a better alternative. Dandelion root tea in moderation is a good alternative to coffee and is excellent for liver cleansing and moving your bowels.

"Water is the most neglected nutrient in your
diet but one of the most vital."

Kelly Barton

Drink pure water

Water is the basis of all life on the planet as well as the most important building block of living organisms. Studies show that drugs entering waste water have an effect on the environment and ultimately you. The quality of your life is connected to the quality of the water you drink.

Water is an easy and economical way to start detoxifying your body. You need 33mls of water per kg of body weight on a daily basis and are likely to need more whilst cleansing. Look into water filters, the best are those that take fluoride and chlorine out. You can also drink bottled water, though think of the environment with all that plastic and avoid BPA in some plastic bottles. Warm water is absorbed into your body more easily but is not good if it has metals in it. Whilst many of you are dehydrated be careful not to over-hydrate because when you do this you will pee out important minerals.

One way of restoring the 'aliveness' in your water is with the plocherwaterkat or echostream water energiser. Another reason to consider a water filter is that some houses have heavy metals that come through the pipes. Lead pipes were used in houses built in Australia before 1939. Lead based solder on brass fittings and copper pipes were used in houses as recently as 1989. Boiling water condenses heavy metals and makes them more absorbable.

You can send a sample of your water to a laboratory for testing if you do not know about your plumbing or see a naturopath who has testing equipment.

Tank water can also be contaminated with lead paint or lead flashing from the roof, microbes and air pollution.

Ozone (03) is a natural, colourless gas with a fresh odour. Nature creates ozone in the air after a storm and this is the fresh smell you notice. Ozone is used to sterilise food, rejuvenate hair, skin, the scalp, for cancer and other medical treatments. Ozone can be made using an ozoniser and adds an extra cleansing quality to water.

Exercise

Exercise greatly benefits the digestion and elimination. It is one of the key factors in preventing constipation. Getting fresh oxygen for your blood and using your lungs is important for healing. Aim to do at least half an hour a day. Whilst you are cleansing avoid strong exercise as you need to conserve energy to cleanse and revive your body. You can do gentle movement like walking, trampolining or use a small lymphaciser (fantastic for detox) yoga, tai chi, swimming in sea water and gentle dance. If you have not exercised regularly, start with 5 minutes daily and build up by 5 minutes a day until you get to 30 minutes a day.

Skin brushing

The skin is the largest elimination organ and is connected to the circulation and lymphatic system (your glands which carry toxins, excess fluid and waste from your cells away from the blood). You make new skin every 24 hours and the health of your skin relates to your blood, lymphatic system and liver.

Skin brushing removes the top layer and helps to release acid waste. The skin needs to eliminate and is usually covered in too many clothes.

Get a pure vegetable bristle brush (do not use nylon) and before you get into the shower each day, brush your skin starting from your feet moving up your body. Brush your entire body (except your face) in any direction. Your skin will tingle a bit at first and as you get used to it you can brush a little harder.

Lymphatic and other massage

Unlike your heart, your lymphatic system doesn't have a pump and relies on movement to get it working. If your lymphatic system is not working effectively, waste and fluid builds-up in your tissues and then the cells can't take up nutrients and oxygen properly. Often your body will swell and the glands, predominately under your neck and groin, will swell. The lymphatic system also helps fight off infections.

When I was working in hospitals, often people who were in a coma or needed a long period of bed rest had lymphatic problems, where their legs and arms would swell with fluid. They had to wear tight stockings, have appliances around their limbs as well as physiotherapy to help pump the lymph. This happened because they weren't moving.

In countries like Belgium, lymphatic massage is prescribed for life for women who have had breast cancer. They have found that those who have it regularly have great survival rates and the cancer doesn't come back.

You also have lymphatic nodes within your digestive system, so any help for your lymph will stop those nodes becoming overloaded.

Using essential oils like lemon, lime, may chang and rosemary help the lymph. You can use a carrier oil like almond oil and for every two millilitres of carrier oil (almond, avocado, grapeseed) add one drop of essential oil and then massage it into your body. So therefore, you can add ten drops of essential oil to twenty millilitres of carrier oil.

Other massages are also beneficial like Swedish, Thai and remedial massage.

Lymphaciser

The lymphatic system runs close to the circulatory system and is vital for transporting wastes and excess fluids away from your cells. It is also important for immunity. A small rebounder or lymphaciser is fantastic exercise for your lymph and moves waste though your bowel.

Zen Chi

This is a little machine that you put your feet in. It rocks your body from side to side. The rhythmic motion massages your whole body and sends energy waves through the body. It's fantastic for constipation, circulation, detox, enhancing lymph drainage, aches and pains and it's profoundly relaxing.

Sunlight

Sufficient sunlight is critical for good digestion. Light on the eye signals the pituitary gland to produce hormones which are essential for the gut. At least 20 minutes of sunlight a day on your forearms and face or equivalent body surface is needed. Vitamin D from sunlight helps happy hormones in the brain. If you feel happy there is less stress on your digestion. Dr. Johanna Budwig has found that "electron rich foods act as solar resonance fields in the body to attract, store and conduct the sun's energy in our bodies." Eating some raw food, getting out in the sun and allowing the sun to reach the eyes by occasionally removing sunglasses will help vitamin D and absorption of vital energy from the sun.

Saunas

Saunas are wonderful for detoxification. It is best to go into a Far Infrared Sauna as these have more power at pulling out toxins like heavy metals. They are more economical and induce 2-3 times more sweat than other saunas and were first developed in Japan. They help pump out toxins at a cellular level rather than through the blood. These saunas pull out toxins that are 1½ inches deep and stored in fat. Pesticides, plasticisers and some pharmaceuticals are man-made chemicals which the body can struggle to get rid of. They are fat soluble and are largely stored in the fatty tissue under the skin. Saunas have been proven to be very effective in removing these types of toxins. As you sweat you will release toxins from your skin and lymph. It is ideal to have one every day during detoxification. Make sure you drink plenty of filtered water to stop dehydration and to replace the water you lose. If you have a medical condition that is affected by heat like high blood pressure, menopause and adrenal exhaustion, avoid saunas.

Ideally stay in the Far Infrared Sauna for 45 minutes if you can, at 50°C. If you exercise beforehand it helps mobilise the toxins even more. These saunas substantially increase lymphatic drainage. Make sure you towel off or shower to prevent toxins reabsorbing.

Drink ½ a litre of water before you go into the sauna and keep up electrolytes lost in sweating with coconut water, or adding a teaspoon of celtic salt to a litre of water or a more pleasant vegetable juice.

Make sure your mineral content is high before and after the sauna e.g. vegetables juices.

Hot and cold showers

These are fantastic for the circulation and to move the lymph. Get under a warm shower then turn it to cold for 15 seconds, it will make you take deep breaths and shiver a bit. Then turn the shower back to warm, then warmer still as long as you can tolerate it. Then go back to cold as you did before. Repeat this until you have done cold five times, finishing on cold.

I have seen amazing recoveries from ulcers and other problems where the circulation is impaired, using hot and cold water. It's very beneficial to do this over your abdomen to stimulate blood flow and help constipation and inflammation. With foot problems (poor circulation/ulcers) it can be done with bowls of hot and cold (which can include ice) water. I know one man who recovered from chronic fatigue by having hot and cold baths every day. His wife bought bags of ice from the petrol station and he'd sit in the cold bath for some time (it stimulates white blood cells which is part of your immune system) then he'd step into a warm shower and repeat the process. It takes a lot of courage to do but some people swear by it. Ice treatment is an age old naturopathic remedy in Europe where people swim in near freezing water in winter for short bursts. I'd avoid it if you have a heart condition.

Epsom salt and bentonite baths

Epsom salts are **magnesium sulphate** and they help toxins move out of the skin as well as relaxing the muscles. Bathing in Epsom salts and/or bentonite clay once or twice a week will help your body with elimination. Bentonite clay draws on toxins like a magnet and is very good for helping to remove heavy metals. Not all clays are the same and Australian clays do not meet purity standards. It is important that the bentonite is calcium bentonite and is very fine with the correct pH. Herbs are best not added to clay but salt and magnesium salts are fine. For these products contact info@ detoxspecialist.com.au

Turn off the phone, light some candles, put on relaxing music and dim the lights. You can add up to six drops of lavender, chamomile and or geranium oils to the bath or into an aromatherapy burner with water for added relaxation. Make yourself a cup of herbal tea or water and lemon juice to sip by the bath. This will create the scene and you can't help but be relaxed.

Add half a cup of salt or clay to a warm bath and relax for twenty minutes. It is best to do this before bed.

If you have psoriasis or eczema you are better with clay.

Epsom salts are very cleansing but bathing in them too often can be depleting so another choice is **magnesium chloride.** This is more nutritive and feeds the body with magnesium and is useful for tired muscles and stress. It has a less cleansing effect than Epsom salts.

Sitz baths

These are small baths with a seat either side. You can put cold water in one side and warm water in the other and alternate sides to stimulate circulation in your lower body. Alternatively you can sit in cold water with your legs out. The impact is on the abdomen so it's effective for digestive problems, especially congestion and reproductive problems.

Castor oil packs

Castor oil penetrates deeply into the skin because of its light molecular weight and as a result tissues and even organs can benefit from its anti-inflammatory properties. It helps the liver, abdominal pain, constipation, detox and improves digestion.

How to make a castor oil pack

Soak a piece of flannel-like material (3 layers of undyed wool or cotton flannel, large enough to cover the area) in castor oil and place it on your tummy. Lie on an old towel.

Cover with a plastic sheet or cling film and then place a hot water bottle on it for 1 hour.

Rinse the skin with a diluted solution of water and baking soda.

Store the pack in an airtight container in the fridge. It may be reused up to 25 times.

A common area to apply the castor oil pack is on the right side of the abdomen, between the upper part of the rib cage and the upper edge of the hipbone. Another common area is across the abdomen from the right to the left side of the body. Application is usually for 1 to 2 hours, approximately 3 times a week.

Place a heating pad on top of the castor oil pack to keep it very warm during application. It is best to consult your health care practitioner to determine the frequency of application. You can use the same castor oil pack for additional applications. It is important to discard the pack after a certain number of uses or when it becomes rancid. It may be helpful to store the pack in a plastic storage container and refrigerate between uses. The wool and cotton flannel packs can be used for approximately 25-30 applications before they are to be discarded.

Coffee enemas work exceedingly well to overcome the inflammatory aches and pains of bowel cancer (and other cancers), arthritis and other painful body degenerations. People with cancer find it amazing for pain relief. The action of coffee rectally is very different from oral ingestion. These enemas remove circulating toxins that overburden the body, by dilating bile ducts (gall bladder) and by cleansing the liver.

Dr. Gerson believes that the liver is our most important organ for maintaining the body's biochemistry for health as well as overcoming degenerative diseases, cancer in particular. Dr. Gerson further found that the cellular systems and body tissues also excrete waste products accumulated over many years from absorbing:

Poor air

Bad water

Food additives and chemicals

Viruses

Germs

and other toxic items.

In order not to overload the liver which filters these poisons out of the blood, he found a way to open the bile duct and help the liver release the body's accumulated poisons by using his renowned coffee enemas. In some cancer patients, Dr. Gerson observed their toxicity to be so severe that he decided to give coffee enemas every 4 hours to detoxify the body.

Dr. Gerson found the problem underlying illness was due to a deficiency of minerals and toxicity. Combining vegetable juices for minerals and enemas speeds up your healing.

Dr. Peter Lechner, M.D. from the surgical division of the Landskrankenhaus in Graz, Austria wrote in a clinical report saying, "Coffee enemas have a definite effect on the colon which can be observed with an endoscope."

Another scientist, Wattenberg, and his co-workers were able to prove in 1981 that the palmitic acid found in coffee promotes the activity of the enzyme glutathione s-transferase many times above the norm. This enzyme is responsible for binding free radicals which the gall bladder can then release.

No other material other than coffee is known to stimulate free radical quenching in such a proportion. The free radicals are mopped up and removed by glutathione enzymes using coffee enemas.

During the time the coffee is held in the intestines, all the blood in the body passes through the liver at least 5 times. The blood circulates through the liver every 3 minutes.

The liver replaces itself every 3 months and the palmitate compounds, caffeine, theobromine and theophylline in coffee cause:

Dilation of the liver's blood vessels and bile ducts.

Relaxation of smooth muscles.

Stimulation of intestinal peristalsis (bowel movement).

Increased bile flow.

Toxic bile is flushed out and along with its bile salts removes waste products of metabolism:

Ammonia

Toxic bound nitrogen

Polyamines

Amino acids

Coagulated clumps

Getting rid of these frees the body from becoming poisoned by its own wastes.

How to do a coffee enema

Make a cup of organic coffee and combine this with tepid water in a 2 litre enema. Hook the enema up in your bathroom and insert the tube using some coconut oil as a lubricant. Lying down insert the mixture until you feel full and then hold it in for at least 10 minutes if you can. It helps to lie on your right side. When you get the urge, go to the toilet and if you have any mixture left repeat this again.

It does take time and can seem overwhelming at first but when you see the benefits it's worth the time and effort.

Note: Coffee has a very different chemical action in the body when you drink it and is not recommended.

Other enemas that are useful: adding to water in an enema bag:

Bentonite clay - 2tbsp. draws toxins out of the bowel and cleaves onto metals.

Garlic - 2 cloves crushed is a natural antibacterial and anti parasitic.

Chlorophyll - 2 tbsp. is a great cleanser.

Aloe vera - ½ a cup helps inflammation and is a mild laxative.

Colonic Cleansing

If you feel like the bottom is coming out of your world have a colonic and the world will come out of your bottom!

There are several options for cleansing the colon which include herbal laxatives, diatomaceous earth, psyllium, bentonite clay, oxygen based cleansers, fibre supplements, enemas, colemas and colonic hydrotherapy. The last 3 are mechanical ways of cleansing the colon using specialised equipment and they are administered rectally.

Regular colon cleansing gives the colon a spring clean and it is also useful for toxic build up on the colon wall and for constipation.

Enemas have been used for centuries and nowadays generally consist of a 2 litre bag for water and a tube which can be easily inserted by yourself at home. The downside with enemas is that they just clean the lower part of the colon but they can be very effective for the relief of constipation. The upside is that a variety of substances can be put into an enema and these can have beneficial effects. Enemas are also very portable and easy to administer. I suggest doing enemas after a colonic hydrotherapy as a colonic cleanses the bowel more thoroughly. By doing this, the substance in the enema can travel further around the bowel and do its job of cleansing e.g. coffee, garlic or chlorophyll.

Colonic hydrotherapy is also known as colonics and colonic irrigation. It's an amazing method of cleansing the whole of the large intestine using purified water. It gently cleanses your rubbish out and is rather like soaking clay off a pipe. It is safe and effective and not nearly as intimidating as it sounds. It is best to have a therapist with you throughout the treatment and for most people it is painless.

Closed method

You are covered up throughout the treatment and a small disposable speculum is inserted into the anus with lubrication; this then attaches to disposable tubing and a glass viewing tube. The colonic therapist then adjusts the water pressure and temperature to suit each individual need, bearing in mind the pressure never goes over a certain marker. In this way the water works with the bowel muscle and water is only put into the person until it meets a blockage or the bowel wants to push material out. Everything is enclosed within pipes, so there is no odour. The bowel is cleansed and the muscles are also strengthened. The water going into the person is separated from the waste matter coming out to avoid contamination. The therapist is with you throughout the treatment giving you abdominal massage and adjusting the machine to suit your needs. This ensures there is duty of care and offers comfort to the client.

The environment is healthy and there are no smells as everything goes out through tubes. The therapist is able to see what comes out and gives feedback information about the client's digestion. The client can also view waste matter leaving their body. In some cases the therapist may ask the client to have stool or other tests done if they suspect something needs attention. The treatment lasts about 45 minutes and afterwards any remaining matter will come out when you are sitting on a toilet. The quality of the treatment depends obviously on the expertise of therapist and the quality of the machine. After trying all the methods of colonics I decided to train in this method as I think it gives the most benefit. I have been practicing and training people in colonics since 1992 and have never seen any grave dangers with this method. You want to be sure that your therapist is well trained, knows when to refer you to a specialist and will not overdo or under do treatments that are needed.

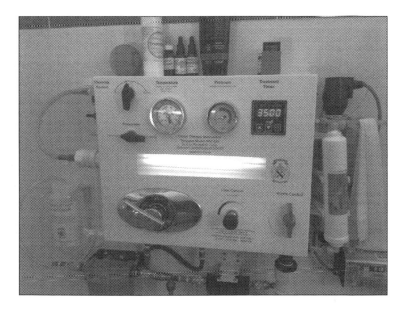

Open method

These are self-service systems and there are a lot of them around. You lie on a small speculum rather like a catheter which inserts into your rectum and underneath you is a type of toilet inserted into the bed where all your waste matter leaves. As the speculum is small it can push into the side of the bowel and occasionally cause problems. All your waste goes around the tube that is in you and down the toilet. As faecal matter is exposed there is odour as there would be if you were on a toilet. You are usually left alone for the duration of the treatment and generally there is not enough duty of care. With this type of colonic treatment, water is always going into you even when you push out, therefore it cannot be catered to individual muscle action and there is a risk of overstretching the bowel.

I find this type of colonic treatment is often overdone and people go for many sessions to relieve a problem which is best helped in part by colonics and in part by other natural treatments that get to the root cause of the problem. However, some people swear by them and the choice is up to the individual. Some people find their bowel seizes with this type of treatment and because there is no one else in the room they keep filling up but can't evacuate and get extremely bloated and uncomfortable. One of my clients went every week for an open colonic to relieve chronic constipation. When she came to me all I did was change her diet and she didn't need a colonic again for a long time. This type of treatment requires minimal qualification, though the therapist may be trained in another modality. It is also cheaper than closed method colonics but there is no one-on-one attention.

Colemas are large buckets that usually hold 20-30 litres of water and they also consist of a board that fits over a toilet. You insert a small speculum into your anus and you have control of how much water you put into your colon. When you want to evacuate you go around the tube that is inside you into the toilet. Various herbs and clay can be added to the buckets. These are common at some health resorts or for self-administering at home. They hold a lot more water than an enema but the principle is similar.

Do these methods strip my bowel of good flora?

Most colonic clinics will give you probiotics after a treatment and often a course of them. Most people have so much rubbish and such an imbalance of good to bad bacteria that they need cleansing to give space for the good bacteria to grow. Like anything, problems can occur if you overdo the treatments and you need an honest therapist who knows what is right for you. In most cases, the benefits are amazing and help restore all over health. It is not recommended for severe haemorrhoids, active inflammatory bowel disease, active diverticulitis, bowel obstructions, low potassium or salt and undiagnosed rectal bleeding.

Whatever type of colonic you choose, I think it's important to also back it up with either naturopathy or Chinese medicine or a similar approach to get a full diagnosis, allowing maximum healing potential rather than symptomatic relief.

Breathing

Breath is the key to life and oxygen is essential for detoxification. Use your lungs and breathe deeply. There are lots of breathing exercises you can do to become more conscious of your breathing and to help you relax. Deep breathing has a powerful effect on your bowel allowing it to relax and heal. A simple one is breathing in for the count of four and out for the count of five for at least ten minutes a day. It's easy to get into this habit when you are stuck in traffic, waiting in a queue or watching T.V. For asthma you can look at Bueteko breathing.

Pregnancy

Detoxification is not to be attempted during pregnancy or breastfeeding however, it is ideal as part of a preconception program. If you fall pregnant while doing a detox, stop the program and contact your health practitioner.

Medication

Detoxification has the potential to change the way some medications work. Discuss this with your health practitioner.

Let's start

The week before you start remove all processed food, caffeine, sugar, animal proteins and soft drinks from your diet. Stick to whole grains, vegetables, salads, chickpeas, beans, lentils and tempeh. If you need animal protein have sardines or salmon. You want to get your body used to whole nourishing foods, take the load off your digestive system and absorb valuable nutrition. Pineapple and pawpaw enhances digestion.

Removing potential toxins allows your digestion to work better as it starts breaking down existing toxins and giving the body a rest also allows time for repair.

Start each day with 2 glasses of water with the juice of 1 lemon. This cleanses your lymphatics, helps your liver and sets up your digestion for the day.

Start implementing the lifestyle advice above: skin brushing every day, having salt baths once or twice a week, saunas, gentle exercise and relaxation.

Fasting has been done all through history by people like Jesus and Ghandi to clear the mind and enhance energy. When the energy is taken away from digestion the body can detox and heal.

After a week of reducing your toxic load, if you are feeling up to it and your pH is about 6.6 you can do a vegetable juice and lemon fast for 3 days, each day taking a teaspoon of psyllium husks and bentonite clay with the juice. This will act as a gentle broom through your intestine and help stop hunger. Mix the juices with 50% filtered water and have lots of green juices. You can include wheatgrass or add a few teaspoons of chlorophyll into juices and drink herbal teas like milk thistle. For 2 days either side of it, eat fresh organic vegetables and lemons, you can also include olive oil, apple cider vinegar and kitchen herbs (see kitchen pharmacy Chapter 11).

A citrus purge (invented by William Kelly) can be very beneficial for high toxicity and weight loss. Consuming up to 12 lemons and 12 grapefruit a day diluted in water and drinking a glass an hour over 5 days can have profound results. It is best to do this under the supervision of an experienced health professional.

Fasting with water only can be harmful as there is no input of minerals from vegetables to mop up circulating toxins which can become highly reactive.

When coming off a detox you want to be careful to stick to wholesome foods. Toxic processed foods will shock your body and start undoing all your good work.

If this is too much you can stick to the following diet for 3-6 weeks making sure you have about 2 litres of water over the day (33mls per kg or body weight) and more if you are having saunas. After a week you can introduce animal protein making sure it is organic.

Adhere to the advice above taking out processed foods and sticking to a clean diet. Eating green vegetables, ricebran, green tea and olive oil helps get rid of organic pollutants. Plan your food well in advance, preferably a week at a time so that you can shop and pack food and choose healthy restaurant food if you eat out.

Introduce fresh herbs mentioned in Kitchen Pharmacy and fermented foods mentioned in ferments. For healthy carbohydrates stick to brown rice, quinoa, buckwheat and millet. These can also be made in a slow cooker and will last a couple of days in the fridge in a sealed container. Have vegetable salads or vegetable juices at every meal.

There are flushes that can be beneficial done under supervision; these include a vitamin C flush, liver/gall bladder flush and colonic hydrotherapy.

Cookware - refer to chapter 4. It is important to use safe cookware especially when detoxing.

Recipes - you can use any of the recipes in Chapter 12 except the deserts and cakes, which are healthy to have when you come off the detox, providing you don't have candida.

It is good to cleanse periodically as toxicity can give you symptoms like fatigue, nausea, headaches, infections, poor memory and concentration, diarrhoea and more serious problems if the toxins are very harmful.

Toxins you may be open to every day

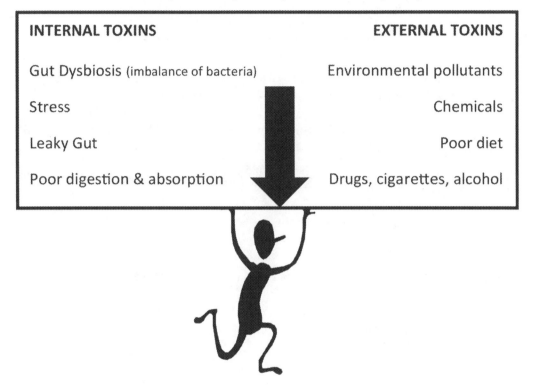

INTERNAL TOXINS

Gut Dysbiosis (imbalance of bacteria)

Stress

Leaky Gut

Poor digestion & absorption

EXTERNAL TOXINS

Environmental pollutants

Chemicals

Poor diet

Drugs, cigarettes, alcohol

CHAPTER 11

Kitchen gut Pharmacy

"Eating everything you want is not that much fun. When you live a life with no boundaries, there's less joy. If you can eat anything you want to, what's the fun in eating anything you want to?"

Tom Hanks

Chapter 11
Kitchen gut Pharmacy

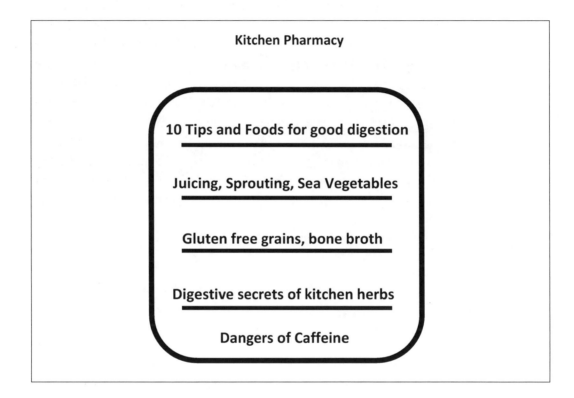

Here are some dietary tips for your digestion and valuable food to use as medicine in your kitchen.

Healthy wholesome food is vitally important for good health, just as much as oxygen and water. It is best to have 50% plant food on your plate and with a variety of colours. The rest of the plate is usually best with 25% protein and 25% carbohydrates. In some cases of chronic digestive illness, grains are best removed.

Different Diets

There is an argument that we should be vegetarian as our DNA is 98% the same as gorillas who are vegetarian. However, mountain gorillas eat ants, snails and grubs (they chew for 6 hours a day) and we are just as closely related to chimpanzees who mainly have a vegetarian diet but they also eat honey, birds and their eggs and small mammals, in particular monkeys, though they may only eat mammals once a month. Often when people become vegetarian or vegan they become a lot more conscious about eating healthy vegetables and their health increases however, over time they are also prone to deficiencies which need to be monitored, especially B12, the lack of which can cause irreversible damage to your nerves and spinal cord. On the contrary, vegetarians can eat a lot of sugar and white flour and be malnourished. Meat eaters can be acidic due to a lack of vegetables and a poor diet but at the same time there are a lot of conscious meat eaters who eat a lot of plant food, are healthy and care about the way animals are reared and killed. Having a healthy balance of natural nutrients and a large amount of plant food is what makes a difference to your health. Whatever you choose, be monitored by a health professional from time to time so they can see how your diet is working for you.

Cravings and binges

There are various reasons you can get cravings which can be an addiction, allergy, a dietary imbalance or an emotional craving.

Addiction: A food can create digestive problems or headaches and other health problems and the symptoms can be relieved by having more of that food e.g. if you stop eating sugar you crave it then eating it again gets rid of the uncomfortable symptoms. Sugar is very addictive and coming off it is like coming off drugs.

Allergy: you often crave or dislike what you are allergic or intolerant to and it causes physical symptoms and sometimes mood changes. It is best to avoid these foods until your gut is healed and then you may be able to tolerate it again. If you are unsure if you are allergic to a food, allergy testing can be performed. See Ch.6 to test yourself.

Cravings: often arise from a dietary imbalance. A craving for sweets and white flour can be caused by eating a diet too high in protein and fat.

- It can also be a sign of protein deficiency where more beans, lentils, fish, eggs or meat are required.

- It can be a sign of a fungal infection as bad bugs in the intestines love to feed off sugar.

- Low blood sugar can also cause sugar cravings and this can be rectified by eating savoury foods every 3-4 hours with adequate protein, fat and healthy carbohydrates.

- Cravings from an acid/alkaline imbalance are strong. Although alkalising foods like salads and fruit are generally positive, too much will cause you to want more acidic foods to balance your body. Without protein and grains (which are healthy acidic foods if eaten in balance), the craving for acid forming sweets will be high.

If you go on a diet that has too much of one type of food and ignores the balance of what your body needs (protein, fat, carbohydrate, vegetables, salad and fruit) it will catch up with you and cause a craving.

Generally speaking:

- If you crave sugar, then have more whole grains and less salt and dairy.

- If you crave coffee, have more vegetables and salads and less meat and sugar. You can use chicory or dandelion to replace the taste, or have green tea for less caffeine.

- If you crave milk, have more leafy greens, brown rice and fish and avoid sugar and fruit. You can use nut milks instead. Just make sure you keep up other calcium foods like tahini, boned fish, almonds and leafy greens.

- If you crave alcohol have more healthy carbohydrates and bitter greens and eat less fat, salt and animal protein. See recipes for healthy drinks.

10 tips for good digestion

1.   Eat foods that are easy to digest.

Eating foods that are easy to digest and combining them well puts less stress on your digestive system. If you overfill your washing machine with thick heavy fabrics it puts a strain on it and it can break. Your stomach doesn't want to be overburdened with food either as it takes a huge amount of energy to digest it.

- Aim to drink in-between meals.

- If you are very sick just have water, soups and vegetable juices as they are easy to digest.

- Vegetables take 30-45 minutes to digest; incorporate green leafy vegetables with every meal and some bitter leaves like rocket and endives as they help your digestion and your liver loves them.

- Beans, grains and other starches take 2-3 hours to digest. Soak them the night before, remove the soak water. The legumes will digest better and stop gas in your belly if you cook them with a kombu stick (seaweed) and/or a little cumin.

- Meat, fish, poultry: Take 3 or more hours to digest. Incorporating lemon, apple cider vinegar and marinating meat with kiwi fruit and or lemon helps these digest more effectively.

- **Apple cider vinegar:** 1-2 tbsp. in 50mls of water sipped with meals helps digestion. Use lemon on lots of foods and in water to help digestion.

2.   Add herbs to your cooking to improve digestion

When you cook different meals think about how you can incorporate the following herbs as they are all digestive aids: ginger, cardamom, cinnamon, coriander, fennel, dill, oregano, thyme, liquorice and aniseed.

3. Eat at regular meal times

It is important to eat regular healthy meals and eat at the same times of day. Eating similar food groups at similar times each day has a regulating effect on your digestive system. Regular healthy meals help regular bowel movements.

4. Be conscious of what you are eating and your portion sizes

Eating too much is the number one cause of indigestion. Your brain signals the feeling of fullness about ten minutes after you are actually full. If you stop before you are full, most likely you will feel full 10 minutes later. Eat with chop sticks or put your knife and fork down between mouthfuls to help you eat more slowly. Use smaller plates and bowls; you can always go back for seconds if you really are hungry. Eat healthy fat with a meal (e.g. coconut oil, avocado, nuts and seeds) or you may feel starving later on and remember 85% of Australians are not eating enough vegetables so add more to your plate.

5. Chew your food completely and avoid talking while you are eating

Your digestion starts in your mouth and chewing makes the stomach's job easier. Avoid bolting down your food. Your stomach is not designed to digest large pieces of food, and you are more likely to get bloating, indigestion and discomfort if you do bolt your food.

6. Drink warm or hot liquids

Ice cold drinks can slow down the digestive process, the digestive muscles contract and water is not absorbed as well. Warm or room temperature water will encourage proper digestion. Drinking too much around meal time will dilute your digestive juices so they are best drunk between meals. Ideally, drink filtered water without fluoride or chlorine and avoid caffeine, alcohol and soft drinks.

7. Relax during mealtimes

Sit down when you eat, have gratitude and be mindful about what you are eating. Avoid reading a book or watching T.V. whilst eating. Rushing meals or eating on the run increases your stress and slows down the digestive process. Create a calming atmosphere when you eat and after you have finished, sit for 10 minutes. Plan time to prepare, cook and eat your meals.

8. Practice good posture

When you slouch you put extra pressure on the digestive organs in your belly. This can cause poor digestion. It is best if you practice sitting with your shoulders back and your chin tucked in. This allows more room for your digestive organs and will help improve digestion.

9. Don't eat late at night

Avoid eating after 7pm as this is when your digestion is weaker. It becomes weaker still every hour after so there is a considerable difference if you eat at 10pm compared to 7pm. At night your whole body needs time to rest and revive. When you eat late at night you don't produce enough enzymes and other digestive juices to digest your food well. The food sits in your stomach and this can disturb your sleep, make you tired and bloated in the morning. It can also make you foggy in the head and grumpy.

10. Take a walk after eating

Increased activity will actually help kick-start your digestive system and raise your production of digestive enzymes. This will lead to easier digestion and less abdominal discomfort. A gentle walk 15-45 minutes after eating for at least 15 minutes will work wonders.

Bitter and sour foods

Those who feel full and bloated shortly after eating may have issues with not digesting food properly. Consuming bitter foods before and during a meal can help your body to get your digestive juices working and get the most out of your meals!

How to include bitter/sour foods into your diet:

- Drink a glass of water with half a lemon before a meal. This can also be done with a capful of apple cider vinegar in 50mls of water sipped during a meal.

- Use apple cider vinegar (or lemon) and olive oil together as a salad dressing.

- Use bitter foods in your meals e.g. rocket, bitter melon, alfalfa, endives, artichokes, dandelion leaves, neem leaves, or any dark green, leafy, bitter vegetable.

Ayurvedic medicine incorporates different tastes for healing. To improve your digestion, include some bitter leaves at every meal. Bitter foods are antibacterial and help the liver which in turn helps detoxify the gut and bitter foods help kill worms and candida. Bitters also help inflammation on the skin often caused by digestive problems. They promote digestion of toxins and remove toxins from the fat and lymphatic system. They are dry, cold and light so if you need warmth, add some ginger and if you need moisture, add plain yoghurt but remember, most toxic guts have too much moisture.

You need a mixture of tastes in your diet. Below is a table that shows the effects of different tastes on your body. Please note: if you overdo any taste you can cause an imbalance. In the west we consume too much salt and sugar and not enough sour and bitter foods which are imperative for a good digestion.

A balance of 6 tastes for health

Taste	Actions	Primary Sources
Sweet	Builds tissues, calms nerves	Fruit, grains, natural sugars and milk.
Sour	Cleanses tissues, increases absorption of minerals. Helps digestion.	Sour fruits like lemons and limes. Yoghurt and fermented foods.
Salty	Improves taste of food, lubricates tissues, and stimulates digestion.	Natural salts like Celtic and Himalayan salt, sea vegetables.
Bitter	Detoxifies and lightens tissues. Stimulates the liver which can help bowel movement.	Dark leafy greens, herbs and spices like dandelion root.
Pungent	Stimulates digestion and metabolism.	Chilli, garlic, herbs and spices.
Astringent	Absorbs water, tightens tissues, dries fats.	Legumes, raw fruit and vegetables, herbs.

Have a look at the back of your tongue; do you notice a coating? If yes, you need fewer damp/moist foods like wheat, dairy and sugar that cause a glue-like substance in your gut. In your home you want to avoid damp in the walls of your house and you also want to avoid it in your body. Bad bugs love a damp environment. Incorporate more bitter, sour and warming foods like greens, lemons, soups, stews and ginger.

Plant some bitter greens in your vegetable garden or in a pot. If you have space, why not plant a neem tree or some dandelion or rocket.

To strengthen and improve digestion

First thing in the morning you can drink this concoction: blend together 4 basil leaves, ½ teaspoon of coriander powder, ½ teaspoon of cumin, the juice of ½ a lemon, ½ a cup of coconut water or coconut milk. If you have constipation you can add 2 tsp. of chia seeds.

Or: Blend 2 cups of soaked almonds with 1 tsp nutmeg, ½ tsp cloves, ½ tsp. cinnamon, ½ tsp. cardamom and stevia to taste.

For bloating, gas and inflammation

2 tsp. barley, 2 tsp. coriander seeds, 2 tsp. fennel seeds, 4 raisins. Put all of these ingredients in a thermos of almost boiling water overnight. In the morning strain and squeeze these ingredients and add a few drops of lemon juice, 2 tsp. aloe vera juice, 2 pinches of turmeric and 2 pinches of cinnamon. If you have candida, avoid the raisins. If you are celiac avoid barley and use slippery elm instead.

Diarrhoea

If you have been suffering from diarrhoea, you will need to replenish your body as you can feel very weak due to the lack of hydration and loss of electrolytes. Coconut water is high in replenishing electrolytes. Sudden and severe diarrhoea needs medical attention.

A congee is a simple rice porridge which is popularly used in Asia. The rice is easy to digest and helps bind your stools. Cook the rice and water in a covered pot for 4-6 hours on a low heat.

You may add a couple of chopped root vegetables for flavour and nutrients. Add some cracked pepper and Celtic salt when serving, as this will also assist in reducing the diarrhoea or have a cup of boiling water with a teaspoon of cracked peppercorns in it. The pepper binds to the cause and stops the diarrhoea quickly.

Note: Table salt is not advisable as it is heated to 700°C and minerals are taken out. An aluminium compound is added to stop caking when the salt gets moist.

Psyllium husks slow down the bowel and help diarrhoea as well as constipation. Address inflammation and parasites/bugs if that is the cause. Diarrhoea can be a way of getting rid of poisons. My grandmother used to take laxatives when she had diarrhoea to get rid of the poison quickly, although when doing this you need to be mindful of losing electrolytes. Common drugs that stop diarrhoea can be handy in awkward situations but will often delay the process of detoxification. With diarrhoea caused by crohn's and colitis, underlying dietary and other causes need to be addressed.

Grated apple with the skin browned and eaten slowly helps diarrhoea.

Constipation - see Chapter 6

Nutrient dense foods

If you are someone who exercises a lot, or you need building up after an illness like colitis, or if you are breast feeding, the following foods are very nutrient dense and beneficial for you. They also make healthy snacks as they are rich in nutrition, rather than having empty nutrition with lots of calories.

Avocado	B vitamins, beta carotene, vitamin E, monounsaturated oils
Chickpeas	Protein, fibre, B vitamins, calcium, zinc, iron
Eggs	Protein, vitamin A, B vitamins and other nutrients
Fish	Protein, zinc, iron, essential fatty acids (omega 3)
Flaxseeds	Essential fatty acids (omega 3) lignans (in seeds)
Kidney, pinto, mung beans, aduki beans	Protein, fibre, calcium, zinc, iron, B vitamins

Lentils	Protein, fibre, B vitamins, calcium, iron, zinc
Tofu/Tempeh	Protein, B vitamins, calcium, iron, zinc
Nuts and seeds	Protein, calcium, iron, zinc, essential fatty acids, vitamin E
Whole grains quinoa, brown rice, buckwheat, millet	Protein, fibre, B vitamins, zinc, iron, magnesium
Blackstrap molasses	Iron, calcium, B vitamins
Coconut milk	Iron, B vitamins, potassium, omega 6

Glycaemic index

Eating foods that are low on the glycaemic index (G.I.) is a key to weight loss and to prevent your pancreas from becoming exhausted which can lead to diabetes. Low G.I. foods have little impact on insulin. Many people overwhelm their pancreas and don't realise it until it fails. Interestingly, William Banting who first discovered G.I. in 1850 restored hearing loss within 12 months by following a low G.I. diet! Adding a fat to a high G.I. food lowers its impact e.g. having coconut oil on a rice cake.

High G.I. foods to avoid

Potatoes, soft drinks, beer, white sugar, white rice, bread, honey, commercial cereals. Interestingly, cooked carrots have a G.I. 3 times higher than raw carrots.

Low G.I. foods to include

Vegetables, whole grains, beans, dark chocolate, meat, eggs, fish, legumes, nuts, seeds, stevia and xylitol (natural sweeteners).

The joy of sprouting

What is sprouting?

Sprouting is growing small seeds, grain or beans like mung been seeds into little living green plants.

The stored nutrient is allowed to burst through with abundant nutrition. The new growth includes the shoot, seed/grain/bean and root, jam packed with nutrition.

- Firstly it increases many nutrients and is easy to digest.

- Calories actually decrease so that's a plus if you are on a weight loss diet.

- The chlorophyll and enzymes increase as the plant becomes a living food. These enzymes help with digestion.

- The B vitamins increase 10 fold, the vitamin C, A, E, K, zinc and calcium increase as well as the protein.

- The fibre and water content are high.

- It removes enzyme inhibitors which can impair digestion; these are known as phytic and oxalic acid.

- It reduces gas producing compounds known as oligosaccharides.

- You will find it is so easy to do and very rewarding and if you are on a budget it's incredibly cheap.

Many years ago when I was travelling and hiking, I made sprouts in stockings hung over my backpack and I watered them as I went past streams. This was not only fun but it was great to have some live fresh food as all the other food during the hikes was dried or tinned.

If you have kids it's a great way to start getting them involved in watching food grow and you don't even need a balcony or a garden! Kids are much more likely to want to try foods they have grown.

What to sprout?

You can sprout a whole variety of seeds, beans and grains. Some take longer than others. Alfalfa is very popular and like other sprouts can be used on salads, mixed with rice after cooking or added to soups after the soup has been cooked.

Here are some ideas and you can find these at your local health food shop or market:

- Mung beans, chickpeas, aduki beans, lima beans, clover, barley, rice, oats, peas, lentils wheatgrass. Wheat grain changes to wheatgrass which you may have had at a juice bar. Broccoli sprouts have the highest number of antioxidants, in particular sulphurophane which is amazing for detoxing in the second phase of liver detoxification. There are 2 phases of liver detoxification that happen every day and they allow you to release harmful chemicals and everyday toxins.

- Pumpkin seeds, sunflower seeds and most grains need to be soaked for 4-12 hours before sprouting. Chickpeas and peas for 12 hours.

Most sprouts only cost 20 cents for a cup. How cheap is that for all the benefits!

How to sprout

There are three ways you can do it:

1. Buy a sprouter from a health food shop. They can be easier when starting out.

2. **Glass jar method**

What you will need:

- A large glass jar with a wide mouth.

- Gauze or cheese cloth to cover the top of the jar.

- A rubber band to hold it in place.

- Fresh filtered water.

- Choose a seed of your choice which can be purchased from a health shop; start with something easy like alfalfa or mung bean, just one type at a time.

Method

1. Add enough seeds to cover the base of the jar.

2. Cover the seeds with about 4 cm's of water.

3. Add the gauze cover and rubber band and secure gauze then pour the water off letting the seeds settle back into the jar.

4. Repeat the rinsing two or three times a day and store the jar in a dark area of your kitchen. For proper drainage the jar is best stored upside down at an angle of 50-70 degrees. An angled dish rack works well.

5. After two or three days shoots will appear and the seeds will require sunlight. Place them on the kitchen bench near a window or on a window sill and continue to rinse twice a day.

6. Depending on the sprout they will be ready anywhere from day three to day six. The sprout will be green with a shoot half a cm long or longer.

7. Remove and store in an airtight container in the fridge to eat in salads, on soups or any way you fancy.

3.   The tray method

What you will need:

• A tray at least 2-3cms deep.

• A high nutrient dirt mix or soaked cotton wadding.

• A spray bottle.

Method:

1. Line the base with dirt mix or soaked cotton wadding.

2. Sprinkle seeds into the tray.

3. Spray water onto the seeds two to three times a day.

When the seeds are ready cut them and store in an airtight container in the fridge to eat in salads, sandwiches, on soups after cooking or on stir fries (sprinkle on after you have finished cooking) or any way you fancy as a healthy snack. Eat them in a few days as they can go mouldy if kept too long.

Tip: If your sprouts ferment and smell whilst growing them make sure you rinse them more often and check to see when they are done.

The wonders of WHEATGRASS

Wheat grass is a powerful, nutrient-dense sprouted food. It is easy to digest and for anyone with a compromised digestion it provides a lot of nutrition. In fact, 1kg of wheat grass is equivalent to 25kg of vegetables. It was actually used a lot many years ago to help vitality and fertility and stopped when supplements were produced in 1930. It became all the rage in 1960 when Ann Wigmore from the famous Hippocrates foundation cured herself of life-threatening colitis. Wheatgrass contains an abundance (70%) of a green pigment called chlorophyll which is essential for all of us.

Wheat grass contains 100 enzymes, 12 vitamins, 21 amino acids and several bioavailable phytochemicals, antioxidants and minerals. Chlorophyll is such an important substance and is almost identical to haemoglobin. It is easily absorbed and increases red blood cells (blood building), cleanses the blood, is a liver tonic and removes debris form the digestive tract. It is also anti-inflammatory, antibiotic and excellent for detoxification, especially for the heavy metal cadmium and for nicotine. Two Nobel prizes have even been awarded for research on wheatgrass. Inflammation is a huge problem in many digestive disorders and C-reactive protein is a great test you can have at a pathology laboratory to check your inflammatory levels.

It doesn't end there, wheatgrass also speeds healing in the gut and is antifungal and therefore good for candida. Dr. Bernard Jensen stated that red blood cells doubled in 2 days after bathing in a bath of chlorophyll and water. If you put ½ a cup into an enema and hold it for 20 minutes it is a highly effective colon cleanser. Wheatgrass contains an anti cancer enzyme SOD which stops cell mutation and it reduces a substance called P4D1 which causes cancer to increase. It is alkalising, high in oxygen which kills pathogens, very good for constipation, boosts digestion and topically it works very well for psoriasis and eczema.

How to sprout wheatgrass

Sprouting wheatgrass is a little different as soil is required.

What you will need:

- 2 cups of wheat grass soaked for 20 minutes.

- A garden tray.

- Organic composting soil.

Method:

1. Fill the tray with soil and spread the seeds evenly on top of the soil.

2. Spray with water twice daily ensuring good ventilation.

3. After 9-12 days your wheat grass will be ready and will be 4-6 inches high.

4. Cut the wheatgrass ½ an inch above the soil, wash it and blend it or put it through a juicer and drink immediately. You only need about 20 mls of wheatgrass for a healthy shot of nutrients.

The advantages of juicing

Have you experienced the freshness and vibrancy of juices? Juicing gives the body live enzymes and bioactive vitamins and minerals. Many people are acidic and need alkalising and vegetable juice and lemon in juice is fantastic for this. Raw juices have been used as a healing agent for many years. The combination of vegetable juices while fasting stimulates the mobilisation of toxins stored in fatty tissue. It slowly releases these and moves them into the blood stream, then out of the body via the liver, kidneys or bowel.

Toxins tend to hide in fat cells as a way of protecting the body, so typically they won't show up in a blood test unless the body has been recently exposed to them. Many of you will have had fresh fruit juices however, I wouldn't recommend these on a regular basis because of the high fruit sugar and the havoc that it can play with your digestion. Many people have fructose (fruit sugar) intolerance and if you haven't you can develop it by consuming too much. High fructose levels require more work from your pancreas to manage your blood sugar. The sugar content in fruit juice stimulates the pancreas to release insulin and this in turn inhibits the growth hormone which slows down tissue repair. If you are going to have the odd one, fill half the glass with filtered water.

Lemons and limes are fine to juice with as they alkalise the body and are sour. Vegetable juices are the most healing particularly green vegetables. Ideas for juicing include mixing three or four of the following: carrot, celery, beetroot, ginger, lemon, parsley and cucumber. Cabbage juice is great for stomach ulcers as it is high in glutamine.

Juicing extracts high amounts of vitamin C. Linus Pauling who did a lot of research on vitamin C extended his life for 20 years, after being very sick, by having 10,000 mg of vitamin C a day. This is a huge amount but it shows you what can be done. It allows your gut to heal by increasing your immunity and it also generates vitamin E and glutathione which are important for digestive health.

3,000 mg a day is healing and the Kakadu plum is the highest natural source of vitamin C you can get. It's native to Australia.

Juicing is great when you decide to do a detox in warmer weather, as an energy boost to the start of the day or to get more nutrition.

Avoid pasteurised juices as they are processed and may contain pesticide residue however, they are a much better choice than a soft drink.

Benefits of juicing

- The nutrients are easily absorbed and assimilated.

- They are great when the digestion is compromised and in the colder months ginger can be added for warmth and circulation. A little warm water can also be added.

- They have high antioxidants and phytochemicals which are protective against cellular damage to the gut and the rest of the body.

- They are easy to prepare.

- Green juices are high in chlorophyll which enhances haemoglobin production and is good for your red blood cells. This causes more oxygen saturation in your tissues which is also beneficial; particularly wheatgrass and barley grass.

- Red, purple and blue juices (like cherries, blueberries and raspberries) are high in anthocyanins and bioflavonoids which actively decrease inflammation in the gut and other tissues in your body.

For ulcers see cabbage juice below.

Benefits of smoothies

I think smoothies are a very rich source of nutrients. They are also filling and fibre rich. They can be made using a blender like Vitamix with 30% fruit (if your digestion tolerates fruit) some water and 70% green leaves. For added fibre you can put chia seeds or flaxseeds into the mix.

Food as medicine

ALOE VERA

This is a great tonic for the liver which aids digestion and neutralises toxins. Aloe vera is a blood purifier and in this way benefits the liver, gall bladder and stomach. It helps inflammation and supports gut immunity and therefore benefits colitis, crohn's and inflammation caused by parasites. For inflammation it works well with turmeric. Aloe vera is also a mild laxative (helping constipation), it stops candida penetrating into the blood stream and helps leaky gut.

BEANS contain lots of oligosaccharides, as do cabbage, cauliflower, brussel sprouts, turnips, onions, garlic and leeks. Many of you may not eat beans because of their gassy effect however, long soaking and discarding the water before cooking gets rid of most oligosaccharides and cooking the beans for longer, until you can mash them, softens the starch and fibre and helps digestion. Sweeter beans such as adzuki, black-eyed peas, lentils and mung beans are probably the easiest to digest and cooking beans with a bay leaf, cumin seeds, fennel seeds or a kombu stick reduces gas.

BICARBONATE OF SODA increases stomach pH (making it less acidic and more alkaline) and instantly helps indigestion and stomach pain. It acts like an antacid. It is very effective in small quantities for alkalising but should not be overused as it can cause alkalosis. As a nurse I have seen patients who require a breathing apparatus due to over consumption of bicarb, though this is very rare. It takes far longer for the body to recover from alkalosis than being too acidic.

Tips: ½ tsp. in water helps indigestion and gets rid of pain within minutes. It is best to take it at least 2 hours after a meal as it can interfere with hydrochloric acid and digestion.

BEETROOT

It is a great bowel cleanser and very good for the blood. It is high in vitamin C and iron. It is naturally sweet and a great natural food colouring and some use it as a hair dye!

In recent studies it has been shown to boost endurance and stamina. The nitrate in beetroot can increase the production of nitric oxide which is:

- A regulator of blood pressure.

- A gate keeper of blood flow to most organs.

- A stamina enhancer via oxygen usage efficiency.

- A weapon against infection, including bowel and stomach infections.

I have seen some people's blood pressure go up due to constipation which can cause pressure on the heart and beetroot is one thing that helps the blood pressure and moves the bowel.

It is also beneficial for those who are convalescing or have suffered exhaustion from inflammatory bowel disease or chronic digestive problems.

How to eat beetroot

Beetroot can be so delicious added to food:

- Scrub it with a vegetable brush to clean it.

- Grate it into a salad; it goes especially well with grated carrot and walnuts.

- Use a cheese slicer and slice into a stir fry near the end of cooking. It's lovely drizzled with olive oil and fresh herbs.

- Roast it in the oven with pumpkin. It takes longer than other roast vegetables so either put it in the oven earlier or chop it into smaller pieces.

- It can be used in cake and muffin recipes.

- Use a small amount in a blender mixed with other foods to change the colour of food for kids.

- It's delicious as a fresh juice. You can mix it with other vegetables or have it on its own, or for a real kick blend it with ginger.

- You can boil it, but I'm not a fan of boiling as it takes more nutrients out than the other methods of eating it.

- Fresh tastes very different to tinned beetroot so don't be put off by past experiences of eating it tinned as there's nothing like eating it fresh.

Please note: When I was nursing, occasionally someone would turn up in casualty thinking they were bleeding from their bowel and bladder only to find out it was the harmless beetroot! Don't get scared when you pee after eating it as it stains urine red and can look like blood; the same goes for your stools.

BITTER MELON

This tropical fruit is about the size of a cucumber which looks like a pendulum and has wart-like bumps all over it. It is very powerful for hypoglycaemia and diabetes and promotes insulin and cell uptake of glucose. It has been used to help haemorrhoids, tumours, helicobacter pylori, salmonella and viruses. Unlike fruit, it is very bitter and is used in savoury dishes. For recipes see Ch.12.

Note: Not to be used in pregnancy or breastfeeding. If you are cold, weak and thin limit bitter foods.

Tips: Juice - Dose up to 50 mls daily, under supervision.

BONE BROTH

Bone broth is an absolutely incredible folk remedy for the gut and I have found its healing effects on the gut lining remarkable. Bone broth has an abundance of minerals (in particular calcium, magnesium, phosphorus and potassium) and cartilage, collagen and bioavailable gelatine.

Gelatine has the unique effect of attracting digestive juices, so when you eat it there is dramatic improvement in digestion and breakdown of food. As well as being a digestive aid it is also a blood tonic and increases calcium absorption. Gelatine in bone broth has been very successful for treating colitis, inflammatory bowel disease, leaky gut and Crohn's disease. It is also very good for detoxification due to the number of minerals in bone broth. Gelatine contains an amino acid called glycine and glycine plays an important role in liver detoxification. The liver is constantly dealing with everyday toxins and has 2 phases of detoxification. Glycine plays a role in the 1st phase and it stops muscle wastage. Incidentally, pregnant women need 10 times the amount of glycine than other women. Chondroitin sulphate in bone broth is good for arteries and arthritis. About 70% of our immune cells are found in the gut and the broth increases these immune cells which helps the body heal. It has the highest level of calcium compared to any other food and it's also renowned for its effects on cartilage and joints in the body. Bone broth has been shown to inhibit the growth of cancer and inhibit the growth of blood vessels that supply cancer cells.

How to make bone broth

You can buy bones from your organic shop or from your local butcher. If you get them from your butcher, usually lamb bones are the least toxic if the animals are not organically reared. Bones are very cheap as they are mostly sold for dogs! You can usually get a bag of bones for only $2. You can also buy fish bones and they are often free from the fishmonger as it's what they discard after filleting fish. It is a good idea to get fish bones with the head on as this contains a lot of iodine which is often missing in our diets and imperative for the thyroid gland. It is also very important for brain development in a growing foetus. You can use fish bones, beef, lamb, chicken carcass and other meats and if you include ribs, feet and knuckles, these have an abundance of nutrients. It can seem a bit gross at first; I shuddered when I got my first fish head but you soon get used to it and when you start to feel the healing effects you'll want to have stock in your fridge all the time. If you cook a roast use all of the bones and left overs for your broth.

1. You will need a large stock pot (saucepan) which is an important pot to have in your kitchen.

2. Put the bones in the stock pot and add cold water until they are just covered.

3. Add 2 tbsps. apple cider vinegar per kg of bones and let this sit for 45 minutes before cooking. The vinegar helps extract more of the good nutrients from inside the bones. Add bunches of herbs like sage, rosemary, thyme and coriander (you can remove them later) and you can also add salt if you like.

4. Double the water and bring the heat to almost boiling then simmer for between 6 hours and 3 days if you have a crock pot. Remove the bones and strain. It will last 5 days in the fridge or you can freeze it.

5. For fish it only requires about 4 hours. The broth will develop a scum on top but you can just take this off with a spoon.

You can have it as gravy, add it to rice, have it as a tea or as a soup. You can add garlic, onion, vegetables and make whatever soups you like with it or add it to stews. Having it on a daily basis, even three times a day will greatly enhance your digestion. I have seen such wonderful changes in people who include stocks in their diets and it's only 20 cents a cup for all that healing nutrition!

There are few foods that are so rich in nutrients and in history there are 5 groups of people who live to 130 years old. The common factor is that all of them ate nutrient dense foods from mineral rich mountains. Now it's unusual to live to that age but eating bone broth is a step in the right direction for longevity.

BRAZIL NUTS

Brazil nuts can aid healing of the gut and prevent and treat cancer, as they are the highest source of selenium and have 30 times more selenium than any other food. No pesticides are used as brazil nuts are not grown commercially. The selenium levels can differ according to soil quality.

BROWN RICE

It is very high in B vitamins and magnesium and therefore good to calm nerves. It is very strengthening and has no gluten. It is a good carbohydrate for diabetics. A handful of raw brown rice chewed as the first food of the day helps expel worms.

How to cook it:

1. Put brown rice and water together in a saucepan with a lid.

2. Use 2 cups water to 1 cup rice. Use high heat and bring it to the boil, uncovered.

3. Put the lid on the pot and reduce the heat to simmer. If your lid has a steam valve, keep it closed.

4. Let the rice simmer for 20 minutes.

5. Turn off the heat and let the rice sit in the covered pot for another 10 minutes.

It lasts a couple of days in a sealed container in the fridge. I often have it for breakfast in winter with a nut-milk, coconut milk, kefir or eggs and spinach.

BUCKWHEAT

The name comes from the Dutch "bockweit" which means "beechwheat" because it's shaped like beechnut and nutty like wheat. It's actually not a cereal or grain, but a fruit seed related to sorrel and rhubarb.

Buckwheat is sold roasted or unroasted. Roasted buckwheat is known as kasha (see chapter 12) in traditional European cooking. This type has an earthy nutty taste - served as an alternative to rice or porridge. Buckwheat in any form is often used as an alternative to wheat and gluten containing grains.

The flour is made from unroasted buckwheat (light and dark) the darker the flour the higher in nutritional status. It is used to make pancakes or soba noodles. It is especially good for gluten sensitive individuals. It is an alkalising "grain" cooked into porridge or made into muffins. It is high in B vitamins, magnesium, bioflavonoids and protein.

Health benefits

Buckwheat is high in bioflavonoids, especially rutin (this extends the action of vitamin C and has a synergistic effect and is a powerful antioxidant) which strengthens veins. It is therefore very good for haemorrhoids along with the pith of citrus fruit. Bioflavonoids protect against capillary damage, improve blood flow, help thin the blood and protect cholesterol from damage. Buckwheat is high in magnesium, it has a large 382 mg in one cup! Magnesium plays a big part in relaxing the bowel muscle making it useful for constipation and irritable bowel. Research has shown that 90% of people are deficient in magnesium and stress is a big factor that makes you excrete magnesium. Lack of it can also cause cramping and spasms in the bowel and if you are a woman make you crave sweets before your period. Protein helps cell repair in the gut and B vitamins help energy and stress levels.

Effects on blood sugar

If you have digestive problems you may have blood sugar issues and can be at risk of developing diabetes which is growing at alarming rates. Buckwheat has been shown to be more effective in lowering blood glucose and insulin than wheat when made into bread. It gives you a feeling of fullness. In a study published in The Journal of Agriculture and Food Chemistry it was found that buckwheat lowers blood sugar by 12-19% when fed to diabetic rats. The component is called chiro-inositol, a substance found to play a significant role in the breakdown of the sugar glucoses and it helps cells communicate.

Allergies

As mentioned earlier, buckwheat contains bioflavonoids which are also potent anti-inflammatory agents and have an anti-histamine like action which may reduce typical allergic reactions.

How to cook/prepare

Buckwheat can be sprouted (see section on sprouting) from hard young seeds. The indigestible coat drops off after sprouting. For porridge, rinse it well and use 1 part of buckwheat to 2 parts of water and cook for 20 minutes. Buckwheat with brown rice flour makes great pancakes; mix 50:50 and add an egg and water to your desired consistency. I often make buckwheat pancakes with just buckwheat flour, egg, water, coconut oil and a teaspoon of cinnamon, which is great for balancing blood sugar.

You can also add cooked buckwheat to soups or stews. Have an adventure in the kitchen and mix it with cooked chicken, peas, pumpkin seeds and spring onions or add it into a salad when cool. As a dessert, mix it with coconut cream/milk and cinnamon.

Tips: The flour is easy to make with a powerful blender. Buckinis which are dehydrated buckwheat kernels are sold in health shops and make a delicious and filling breakfast cereal.

CAFFEINE

The advantages of caffeine are that it can make you go to the loo, wake you up and burn fat however, it comes with a much bigger downside.

According to the food standards of Australia and New Zealand and the National Foods Tea Centre Sydney, caffeine can prevent pregnancy, cause miscarriage, increase stress and lead to heart disease. Guidelines in pregnancy are 200 milligrams or less a day. Caffeine increases inflammation in the gut, irritates the bowel and contributes to irritable bowel syndrome and affects digestive juices negatively; it is acidic, causes heat in the stomach contributing to ulcers and it affects the nerves of the whole gut. It stimulates adrenaline and cortisol which in excess can make you a nervous wreck and it decreases immunity.

It raises bad cholesterol and homocysteine leading to heart problems; 5-10 cups a day can cause a heart attack and as constipation puts pressure on the heart, those with chronic constipation are more susceptible. It reduces mineral absorption when taken with or near to a meal. Both calcium and the polyphenols in coffee and tea reduce iron absorption.

Strength of caffeine per cup - 600mg daily is considered safe for adults but far less is advised if you are anxious, stressed, have insomnia or a gut problem. With most gut problems caffeine is best left out of the diet altogether. Some people can handle small amounts of green tea which has beneficial antioxidants. Caffeine is very dehydrating and water is necessary for a healthy bowel movement; clearing toxins and many metabolic processes are dependent on water.

Percolated Coffee 60-120mg per 250mls cup

Black tea 10-50mg per 250ml cup

Green tea 8-36 mg per 170ml cup

Oolong tea 12-55mg per 170ml cup

Cola drinks 48.75mg per 375ml can

Cocoa/hot chocolate 10-70mg per cup

Dark chocolate (cacao nibs have more) 40-50mg per 55g

Energy drinks 80+mg per 250ml cup

Guarana (a herb) is high in caffeine and dangerous for children

COCONUT OIL

There has been a bit of controversy over coconut oil as some people think it is bad for your cholesterol, this is because some studies done years ago were done on hydrogenated coconut oil which is bad news to start with.

Now there is so much evidence that this is a wonderful health food for most people. Dr. Mary Enig is one of the world leaders in research for coconut oil and has promoted it as a food for weight loss in her book Eat Fat, Lose Fat.

If you have ever been to the tropics you may have experienced the deliciousness of a fresh coconut straight from a palm tree.

Coconut oil contains lauric acid which is very beneficial for your immune system and mystiric acid which is anti-fungal and therefore helpful in cases of thrush or candida.

You may think coconut oil is fattening because it is made of saturated fat but unlike cheese that is a saturated fat with long chain fatty acids it has medium chain fatty acids that burn energy quickly. If you eat up to a tablespoon of coconut oil before a meal you will eat far less food so it is good for weight loss. For some of you, this may be too much so start with a teaspoon. It stops your appetite and desire for sweets.

It's also wonderful as a moisturiser.

CUCUMBER

Headache/hangover - Eat a few cucumber slices before going to bed and wake up refreshed and headache free.

Cucumbers contain enough sugar, B vitamins and electrolytes to replenish essential nutrients lost from the body, keeping everything in equilibrium, avoiding both a hangover and a headache.

Snack/binge - Looking to fight off that afternoon or evening snacking binge? Cucumbers have been used for centuries for quick meals to get rid of hunger.

Mouth freshener/bad breath - Don't have mints? Take a slice of cucumber and press it to the roof of your mouth for about 30 seconds for fresh breath. The phytochemicals will kill the bacteria in your mouth responsible for causing bad breath.

EGGS

They are full of nutrition and are tolerated by most people but if you are intolerant, allergic, vegan or find them difficult to digest, these make good substitutes.

What can you eat?

- Egg replacer from health food shop - follow directions on box.

- 2 tbsp. corn-starch = 1 egg

- 2 tbsp. arrowroot flour = 1 egg

- 2 tbsp. potato starch = 1 egg

- 1 banana = 1 egg in cakes

- 1 tbsp. milled flaxseed and 3 tbsp. water = 1 egg. Light, fluffy cakes!

- 1 tbsp. ground chia seeds and 3 tbsp. water = 1 egg.

GLUTEN

If you have digestive problems you may need to avoid gluten which includes: wheat, oats, rye, barley, triticale and spelt. Beer, couscous, breadcrumbs, durum, hydrolysed wheat protein, pasta, semolina, grain vinegar, wheat germ and liquorice lolly sticks contain gluten. Avoid thickeners in foods as most of them contain gluten; they are represented by numbers like 1400 on food packets.

With severe digestive problems all grains need to be removed.

What can you eat?

Rice, quinoa, amaranth, corn, millet and buckwheat

HONEY

It is one of the oldest food preservatives and was used to treat infections before antibiotics were introduced. Honey is the only food on the planet that will not spoil or rot. It will do what some call turning to sugar. If this happens sit the honey container in hot water, turn off the heat and let it liquefy. It is then as good as it ever was. Never boil honey or put it in a microwave as it will kill the enzymes in the honey. You are best to buy cold pressed organic honey as most commercial honey has been heat treated.

Honey has a high sugar content and kills most bacteria. Natural airborne yeasts cannot become active in it because the moisture content is too low. Natural, raw honey varies from 14% to 18% in moisture content. As long as the moisture content remains under 18%, virtually no organism can successfully multiply in honey. However, infants need to avoid honey as their gut is immature and honey can contain spores of Clostridium Botulinum. This can be dangerous as their gut can allow the endospores to transform into toxin producing bacteria leading to illness and even death.

Manuka honey has the highest therapeutic use and is useful for bowel inflammation and bacterial gut infections. I wouldn't recommend honey if you have yeast infections, candida or insulin problems. The quality of Manuka honey is graded UMF (unique Manuka factor) and a number usually from 10-20. The higher the UMF the more antibacterial strength the honey has.

Bees are vital as they pollinate crops. Over the last few years colony collapse disorder has occurred in several countries. The bees disappear from their hives; research has shown that mobile phones interfere with their navigation. Other studies show that genetic engineering also confuses bees.

Peptic ulcers - ½ tsp. honey 3 times daily on an empty stomach.

Upset stomach - ½ tsp. honey taken with ½ tsp cinnamon powder cures stomach ache and also clears stomach ulcers from the root.

Gas - According to studies done in India and Japan, if honey is taken with cinnamon powder the gut is relieved of gas.

Indigestion - Cinnamon powder sprinkled on two tablespoons of honey taken before food relieves acidity and even helps digest heavy meals.

Bad breath - In South America people gargle with one teaspoon of honey and cinnamon powder mixed in hot water first thing in the morning, so their breath stays fresh throughout the day.

CABBAGE juice - has been very well documented for healing peptic ulcers and, more recently, evidence shows it goes well beyond ulcers. It was first observed in the late 1940s and 50s and later research showed the high glutamine content was therapeutic. Glutamine also helps heal a leaky gut. Cabbage juice is also high in indoles and indole 3 carbinol is found to have a role in protecting against the development of breast cancer. It helps the liver detoxify and removes carcinogens from the body.

It is powerful for many gastrointestinal conditions and if you are suffering from an inflammatory bowel you will find this juice gives you substantial relief. Cabbage juice also helps produce gastric juice, helps blood sugar levels and is antibacterial. It inhibits the growth of nasty bugs like candida and parasites and it also quenches free-radicals and slows tumour growth.

CHERRIES- have ellagic acid, a plant phenol which is anti-carcinogenic and antioxidant. Cherries help pull uric acid out of the body and are useful when digestion has become too acidic and gout has developed.

KUDZU (see Ch.6)

LEMON/LIME is highly antiseptic and fantastic for digestion especially if you have overeaten fat or protein. It breaks down mucus and helps parasitic infections. It benefits the liver by stimulating bile formation. It helps indigestion and cleanses the lymph and blood. Lemons break down nasty bacteria in the intestines and mouth and are a good as a breath freshener. Lemon peel has a strong beneficial action on the liver. For digestive help start with 1-3 lemons a day for a week and increase it to 9-12 a day if you tolerate them well and need their properties.

Meat digests a lot better if you marinate it in lemon juice the night before. Lemon also helps digest cooked meat.

MILK

Casein, the protein in cows, sheep and goat's milk and lactose, the milk sugar, can cause problems in some people with digestive disorders. Whilst goat's and sheep's milk are far easier to digest, sometimes these also need to be removed from the diet until the digestive system has recovered. If milk can be tolerated it is best unpasteurised and organic.

What can you eat?

Nut and rice milk. Bear in mind these don't always have the same calcium content as milk so eating foods like green leafy vegetables, tahini, sardines and seaweed is important to meet calcium requirements. Yoghurt and kefir are usually tolerated by the lactose intolerant so these are also good calcium options. Animal milk is often tolerated if it is unpasteurised, raw, uncontaminated and the highest quality milk from cows or goats. Whey milk or cheese is rich in vitamins and minerals. In soured milks (like kefir or lassi) the milk sugar (or lactose) has been changed into lactic acid which is beneficial.

Please note: soy milk can cause hormonal problems and disrupt the thyroid gland. Soy foods are healthy if they are fermented.

Ingredients:

1 cup of soaked (overnight or for at least 4 hours, remove soak water) almonds or cashews or sesame seeds or cooked brown (healthier) or white rice or oats. You can be creative and blend different nuts.

3 cups of pure filtered water. You can alter the water to the consistency you like.

Optional to add in: 2-4 medjool dates or 2 tsps maple syrup, stevia, yacon syrup or rice syrup. 1 tsp. vanilla extract (fresh-cut bean, sliced lengthways and scrape the beans from the pod. 1-2tbsps. carob powder for a chocolate flavoured milk.

Spices that taste nice and are also great for digestion: cinnamon, allspice, cloves and cardamon (this is delicious with cashew milk).

Place ingredients into a high speed blender until mixed well. I love my Vitamix for this.

If you like it smooth, squeeze it through a cheese cloth or a nut-milk bag or you can drink it with the pulp though it will have more texture. Let cooked rice (cook it with vanilla bean) cool for at least ½ an hour before straining.

OATS are best soaked or cooked as this makes them easier to digest and helps negate phytates which can stop mineral absorption. They reduce glucose absorption and therefore help blood sugar. They keep you full and studies have shown that oat eaters ate fewer snacks and less at lunch when oats were consumed at breakfast instead of commercial cereal. Oat bran is high in soluble fibre and just need to be mixed with boiling water. Oats help calm the nervous system and are soothing for the digestion.

Note: Oats contain small amounts of gluten and are not suitable if you are celiac.

Tips: Serve with butter and salt or coconut milk and goji berries or stewed fruit and seeds. You can thicken soups and stews with them.

ONIONS increase digestive juices and help stop bleeding e.g. if you have haemorrhoids. They reduce the risk of colon cancer and increase insulin production. Red onions have more antioxidants. Onion juice (ltsp. a day) is powerful for eliminating worms especially in children. If you don't have a juicer soak 2 sliced onions in half a cup of water for 3 hours and drink the water over the day. Onion juice also eliminates lice and stops hair falling out. Some people are sensitive to the sulphur or fructose in onion and can't eat them.

PAWPAW, a secret for erasing parasites

Orange pawpaw/papaya is full of goodies. The leaves stems and bark have more vitamin A than carrots; the fruit has 80% more vitamin C than oranges and more lycopene than tomatoes. Pawpaw contains the most powerful digestive enzyme papain and a pain relieving compound. Under-ripe pawpaws and the seeds are rich in papain which helps digestion.

Pawpaw helps constipation and releases mucoidal plaque in the intestines. The seeds and under-ripe pawpaw (it has a better effect if it is soaked (peeled) in apple cider vinegar for a day) are very effective for killing intestinal worms. Just grind 20 pawpaw seeds, mix them with water and a bit of rice syrup or other natural sweetener then eat them on an empty stomach for 4 days in a row to help kill worms. You can make a tea from the leaves which is very good for cancer.

If you live in the right climate it only takes 10 months to grow a tree and then you have all that beautiful healthy fruit to eat.

PINEAPPLE

Contains the enzyme bromelain, which aids digestion and helps destroy worms. Pineapple helps diarrhoea and indigestion.

Note: Avoid if you have a peptic ulcer.

POTATOES a healing remedy

Potatoes were originally from Peru and used raw for indigestion, alkalising and inflammatory pain. Russian folklore suggests that all those over 40 should grate a raw potato and eat it daily before breakfast to clear arteries and increase blood flow to the heart. This can in turn help the blood flow to the intestines. When I was walking in Peru, porters used raw potato on muscle pain. It cooled the skin, got rid of pain and absorbed acid from the body.

Note: Cooked potatoes are very high in starch and can raise blood sugar. They are not recommended cooked but a little raw or in juices is alkaline and beneficial.

QUINOA

This is a healthy gluten free grain packed with nutrition. It is has the highest protein content compared to any other grain and is a complete protein. It is high in iron, calcium, B vitamins and vitamin E. It comes in different colours: red, white and black. It can be cooked and used like rice.

SEA VEGETABLES

Seaweed is highly alkalising and nutrient dense so it's good to know how to use it, where to buy it and to start experimenting with this incredible food source. Seaweeds are high in minerals especially calcium, iron, zinc and iodine. They contain vitamin A, C and B vitamins. Seaweed is detoxifying and has an amazing ability to pull out heavy metals from the body like mercury, lead and aluminium. For those on a dairy free diet, seaweed is one alternative for calcium. It is a very good food to add if you have a debilitating gut condition and you need more nutrition.

NORI is the seaweed you may be most familiar with. When you buy sushi rolls or California rolls, nori is what they are wrapped in. You can buy nori sheets from health shops and sometimes the Asian section of supermarkets and Asian grocery stores. When you buy it at a health food shop you can be sure it comes from more healthy seas. If you are new to seaweed, nori is the easiest to use along with dulse. I have found nori is very popular amongst kids especially with a bit of soy sauce. It comes in sheets and you can break these sheets up and eat them plain or you can tear bits up and add them to soups or salads. You can make your own California rolls or cook brown rice and veggies (you can add fish or meat) and lay some on one side of the seaweed and then roll it up like a mountain bread sandwich. Just moisten the edge with water to make it stick and eat it!

DULSE is a Celtic seaweed and usually sold in a shaker a little larger than a salt shaker. It's easy to use as you can just sprinkle it onto anything, fish, salads, soups and rice dishes.

HIJIKI is seaweed that comes in fine strands and has a strong pungent flavour. In Japan it is renowned for making women's hair thick and shiny. It needs to be soaked and bulks up 5 times its original size. It's very good in a salad and can be used in many other dishes.

ARAME needs to be soaked for 10 minutes before eating. It comes in strands and is slightly sweet. It can be added to soups, stews, muffins, pancakes and salads. It's known for its immune boosting qualities which are needed for bowel infections and infestations.

WAKAME is eaten regularly by Japanese pregnant women for its nutrient content. The leaves need to be cut into strips as they expand when cooking. It is also known as sea mustard and is very high in omega 3 fatty acids which are good for bowel inflammation. They go well with sardines, soups and salads, in particular cucumber.

KOMBU comes in long wide sticks. The sticks are good when added to soups and they can be cut into 5cm strips. If you suffer with gas from eating lentils and beans, just add a kombu stick whilst you are cooking and then remove it at the end. It will relieve the problem. It is high in glutamic acid which is good for memory and aids digestion. It also flavours and adds minerals to stocks.

SLIPPERY ELM helps all types of intestinal inflammation or irritation and those with a compromised digestive capacity. It also protects the stomach from erosion or aspirin induced ulceration. It helps with diarrhoea and constipation. Its slimy gel is soothing and calming to the gut wall, allowing repair and protection.

SUGAR SUBSTITUTES

It is in so many commercial foods and it's addictive. Sugar from the cane is full of fibre and is slowly absorbed. Refined sugar is the worst food you can eat. Avoid commercial cereals, sauces, cakes and biscuits.

What can you eat?

Eat more protein and healthy fat like coconut oil to curb your need for sweets. Better alternatives, if you need them, are xylitol, stevia, coconut sugar, yacon syrup, coconut nectar and rice syrup.

YEAST

Although nutritional, yeast is full of B vitamins it can cause havoc if you have bad bacteria or fungus in your gut. Moulds and yeast can feed the fungus and they are found in breads, beer, wine, vegemite, vinegar (apple cider is o.k.), sauces, crackers and some cheeses.

What can you eat?

Yeast free breads, yeast free crackers such as rice cakes or ryvita. For alcohol use gin and vodka as they don't contain yeast. You can use bicarbonate of soda and baking powder in recipes that require yeast for rising.

UMEBOSHI - alkalising plums

These remarkable plums originated in China over 4000 years ago. They are renowned for their alkalising and medicinal qualities. They are small pink and salty and you'll find them in Japanese grocery shops and health shops. They are absolute gems. They stimulate the digestion and help eliminate toxins from the body. They purify the blood and help the kidneys and liver expel toxins. They are also antibacterial, antiseptic and high in vitamin C.

If you have indigestion, have overeaten or have morning sickness these little plums will help. They are high in minerals and protein. You only need 1 plum a day. If you have a strong palate you can chew on an Umeboshi plum, otherwise cut it and serve it with dishes like rice or fish. You can use a nut cracker to crack the pip inside. Within this is an edible seed that tastes like marzipan and is rich in minerals.

Kitchen herbs and spices to include in cooking and teas to help your digestion

ANISEED is used to expel wind and has a mild antiseptic action on the gut.

Tips: add to sweet dishes, curries and teas.

ASAFOETIDA reduces the growth of harmful microbes in the gut, has a laxative effect and it reduces spasms and wind.

Tips: It is available from markets and Indian shops. It is used in Indian cooking and goes well with turmeric. It can be used instead of garlic and onion and tastes like leeks. A pinch with lentils helps with digestion.

BASIL is from the same family as mint. It contains an abundance of flavonoids and volatile oils which protect the body and studies show it helps radiation damage. It is rich in carotenoids which protect the lining of blood vessels from damage. Basil is high in magnesium which relaxes the bowel. It is useful in gut infections and studies show it restricts e. coli, listeria, staphylococcus aureus and other nasty bacteria. It is anti-inflammatory and useful for inflammatory bowel conditions along with turmeric, sage and liquorice.

Tips: Blend with most foods, meat, fish, pesto, salads, (especially tomatoes) and rice. If you cook it, add it during the last 10 minutes to retain the nutrients.

BAY LEAF is from the same family as cinnamon, cassia, sassafras and avocado. It is a very good digestive aid. It is astringent which means it helps contract tissues in the body. It helps relieve gas.

Tips: It works well in soups and stews and is best removed before serving.

BLACK PEPPER stimulates the taste buds and helps to increase hydrochloric acid in the stomach which helps digestion and absorption of nutrients. It is therefore helpful for those who have a poor appetite and are cold. It contains vanadium which is useful in glucose control in small amounts.

Note: Avoid it if you have a gastric ulcer.

Tips: In small amounts it works well in most dishes with salt: eggs, fish and meat. Avoid it if you are overheated.

CARAWAY has a long traditional use for soothing stomach complaints.

Tips: It works well in stews, curries, sweet dishes, pancakes and flat breads.

CARDAMOM helps breaks down gallstones. It helps in constipation, dysentery, and other digestive problems. Interestingly, it's an antidote to scorpion venom.

Tips: It works well in sweet and savoury dishes. Cardamom can neutralise the toughest breath odour. A teaspoon of powdered cardamom added to coffee is delicious. It also blends well with nut milks as a warm drink.

CAROB POD usually comes as a powder and is a good alternative to chocolate. It is high in magnesium which helps relax the bowel muscles making it easier to pass stools.

Tips: It is naturally sweet so no sugar is necessary; you can add it to your favourite milk for an alternative to chocolate.

CAYENNE

Pain relief - cayenne is rich in salicylates a natural aspirin-like compound, increasing circulation which is its most prominent attribute.

Cayenne helps stop bleeding and does not burn. It fights internal bacteria, relieves gas, and helps the action of digestive enzymes.

Tips: Eating cayenne at breakfast decreases appetite and leads to lower fat and calorie intake throughout the day. Cayenne helps boost your metabolism and induces the body to burn off more fat instead of storing it in the body. Add small amounts to soups and stews. Blend a pinch with pineapple and a touch of virgin olive oil for a healthy morning drink.

CELERY SEED has been shown to help inflammation, fluid retention, bacteria, gas/wind. It is good for digestive upsets, including indigestion. It's also great for the urinary tract and joints.

Tips: It goes well with eggplant, fish, butter beans and peas.

CINNAMON has been used for many years as a healing agent. It has essential oils which help significantly with blood sugar problems and type 2 diabetes. It helps the body's ability to respond to insulin. Studies have shown that less than ½ a tsp. of cinnamon per day reduces blood sugar levels in type 2 diabetes. It has been shown that ¼ to ½ a tsp. per day drops blood sugar by 20% and reduces cholesterol and triglycerides in those with type 2 diabetes.

Tips: Cinnamon works well with smoothies, yoghurt, porridge, curries and stews. It has also been shown to help memory.

CHILLI has been shown to kill cancer cells and has an anti-ulcer protective effect on stomachs infected with H. Pylori. Red chillies are high in vitamins C, A and B6. They help lower blood sugar, increase bowel movements and lower pain in I.B.S.

Tips: Chillies need to be eaten in moderation. Never swallow a chilli whole or take them after anal-fissure surgery. They may aggravate haemorrhoids.

CORIANDER (cilantro) like many spices, contains antioxidants, which can delay or prevent the spoilage of food seasoned with this spice. Both the leaves and seeds contain antioxidants, but the leaves have a stronger effect. It is a strong digestive aid and is anti inflammatory. Chemicals derived from coriander leaves have antibacterial activity against Salmonella choleraesuis.

Coriander has been used for the relief of anxiety. Coriander seeds are used in Indian medicine as a diuretic (getting rid of fluid) by boiling equal amounts of coriander seeds and cumin seeds, then cooling and consuming the liquid. They help expel gas and strengthen the digestive system.

Coriander has been documented as a traditional treatment for type 2 diabetes. A study on mice found coriander extract had both insulin-releasing and insulin-like activity.

Coriander increases the creation of bile by the liver.

Coriander is fantastic as a detoxing agent for chelating heavy metals, even helping pull out lead from bones, studies confirm this. Many people have mercury, aluminium, lead and cadmium at toxic levels. This is best analysed with a professional hair analysis.

Tips: The following pesto is very effective for heavy metals and is a digestive aid: use as a spread, dip or sauce.

CORIANDER CHELATION PESTO

- 4 cloves garlic (immune boosting, antiseptic, anti-parasitic)

- 1/3 cup Brazil nuts (selenium, magnesium)

- 1/3 cup sunflower seeds (cysteine)

- 1/3 cup pumpkin seeds (zinc, magnesium)

- 2 cups packed fresh coriander (vitamin A)

- 2/3 cup of flaxseed oil (omega 3)

- 4 tablespoons lemon juice (vitamin C) - use ripe lemons

- 2 tsp. dulse powder (Asian produce stores – seaweed detoxes heavy metals)

- 1/2 cup colloidal silica gel (Planet Health, optional)

- Sea salt to taste

Method

1. Process the coriander and flaxseed oil in a blender until the coriander is chopped.

2. Add the garlic, nuts and seeds, dulse and lemon juice and mix until the mixture is finely blended into a paste.

3. Add a pinch of sea salt to taste and blend again.

It is best stored in dark glass jars if possible. It freezes well, so if you purchase coriander in season and fill jars to last through the year it will make your life easier.

CLOVES are a great source of several vitamins and minerals including manganese, vitamin C, calcium and omega 3 fatty acids. Cloves help expel gas from the intestines, they increase hydrochloric acid (helps digestion) in the stomach and improve the wave-like action of the bowel causing faeces to move; this is known as peristalsis. Cloves are also a natural anti parasitic especially for killing parasite eggs. Cloves warm the stomach and bowel. Clove oil applied to a cavity in a decayed tooth or chewing cloves, relieves toothache. When boiled with water they make a good antibacterial mouthwash. Avoid clove oil on the skin as it can burn unless diluted. It can cause excessive saliva.

Tips: Add to any curry. For a chai tea it blends well with cinnamon, cardamom and ginger. It works well in desserts with stewed apple, pear or rhubarb.

CUMIN is a rich source of iron and has been used traditionally for the gut. Cumin stimulates the secretion of pancreatic enzymes, necessary for effective digestion and absorption.

Tips: Adding the seeds to lentils, beans, cabbage, cauliflower, brussel sprouts, turnips, onions and leeks stops the effect of oligosaccharides in these foods that causes embarrassing gas/wind. The seeds go well in curries, stews and with grains. They blend well with coriander and cumin.

CURRY LEAF is anti-microbial, anti-inflammatory, high in iron and has been shown to reduce liver cancer.

Tip: It is best to cook with onion in the first stages of cooking a curry. It is also delicious in a variety of soups and blends especially well with pumpkin or peas.

DILL The seeds are stronger and the leaves have a soft sweet taste. It activates a nutrient glutathione. This helps protect against carcinogens. It is also effective for weight loss.

Tips: It is good to use for flavouring when fermenting vegetables. It is delicious with fish, chicken and in soups.

FENNEL SEEDS are warming, sweet, calm the stomach, stop spasms in the intestines, relieve wind and stimulate your digestion. They have a protective effect on the gastric lining in relation to ulcers.

Tips: Chew on a few at the end of a meal for easier digestion; it's also great as a tea.

FENUGREEK has been traditionally used in Ayurvedic medicine for diabetes and obesity. Research shows it stabilises blood sugar as effectively as some drugs and it helps insulin resistance.

Tips: It works well in curries and as a tea.

GALANGAL is an Asian root similar to ginger but has a stronger more pungent taste. It has been used in traditional medicine with lime juice as a tonic for the digestion. You can get it from Asian grocery stores and it has a slight pink hue. It can be used like ginger and is good for nausea.

Tips: There are many ways to use galangal; slice it thinly and use it to flavour salads, soups and stews, or grind it and use it in curry pastes and sauces. It tastes especially good with seafood.

GARLIC helps lower blood sugar levels, enhances the body's production of insulin and is therefore useful in diabetes. It also helps yeast, bacterial and fungal (like candida) infections. It is warming, improves digestion and enhances the body's absorption of food. It helps eliminate toxins found in the body and inhibits the growth of different bacteria. It contains allicin, an antimicrobial which helps get rid of parasites and viruses and fights infection. It improves blood sugar issues and helps the body detox from various substances including heavy metals. There are more than 1800 studies on the positive health effects of garlic. There are over 205 published papers that show it has anti-cancer effects. It shrinks tumours and is excellent for preventing stomach and colon cancer.

2-3 cloves a day is a therapeutic dose. Crush the cloves and leave them sitting for 10-15 minutes to allow the therapeutic compounds to fuse together.

Tips: You can crush it in a garlic crusher with the peel on. Garlic enhances the flavour of all dishes including salad dressings and dips. In some people it causes wind/gas and can be replaced with asafoetida. Cooking it for more than 20 minutes above 100°C causes it to lose its potency so add it to food in the last 20 minutes of cooking to keep its precious medicinal qualities. Having garlic and brazil nuts regularly is one good defence against bowel cancer. Brazil nuts are high in selenium, an important antioxidant for fighting cancer. Eating parsley stops bad breath caused by eating garlic. Breast feeding mothers who eat garlic may find it gives their babies colic. Don't take garlic if you are on blood thinners; it also enhances the effects of aspirin (you may need to reduce the dose) and antibiotics.

GINGER is a root that is well known for its beneficial effects on the gut and is a universal medicine. It is excellent at warming, calming, soothing the gut and stopping spasms. It relaxes the intestines and is very good for irritable bowels, motion and morning sickness, nausea, vomiting and weight loss. It warms the digestion and helps strengthen it. It has antioxidant and anti-inflammatory properties and is protective against cancer along with turmeric. Studies show that ginger can reduce colon cancers by 50%. Fresh ginger contains more of the anti-inflammatory gingerol than dried ginger. Dried ginger contains more of the pain killing compound known as shogaol. It is also very good for immunity, circulation and is protective against parasites. Studies also show it helps blood sugar.

Note: Do not exceed 4g if you are on blood thinners or 2g a day in pregnancy and be cautious if you have a peptic ulcer, reflux or gallstones.

Tips: Use dried ginger for stomach pain. Use fresh ginger for vomiting, diarrhoea and cold feelings in the body. You can chop a teaspoon of fresh ginger for tea and for added digestive benefit add some mint leaves. You can juice it and add it to many dishes when cooking.

KAFFIR LIME/LEAVES are used in Thai cooking in pastes and sauces. The fruit, rind and zest can be used.

The leaves can be shredded finely and used in fish cakes, in soups and sauces. They can also be used in a salad. You can put them in a jar of rice syrup for flavour. They can also be added when cooking rice. The juice from the lime is effective for gas/wind pain and indigestion. The leaves are good for the gums. The trees are easy to grow in Australia.

Tips: First remove the central rib in the leaves and you can freeze them in bulk. They work well in curries with chillies, galangal, garlic, ginger, lemon grass and Thai basil. If you use the whole leaf, remove it after cooking.

LEMON BALM (Melissa) is very calming to the gut and helps stops spasms. It is a mild sedative and helps memory. It's great as a tea.

Tips: It can be added to fish and vegetables. The leaves are good in salads and sauces and it's also good for meat stuffing.

LEMON VERBENA has oils that have some antioxidant and antibacterial properties and has anti-candida activity (a fungus that can become opportunistic when immunity is compromised and causes infection). It eases colic and helps digestion after a meal. It is antispasmodic to the gut and therefore good for irritable bowels. It strengthens the nervous system which helps stress that is often associated with bowel problems.

Tips: It is easy to grow in the garden and makes a very refreshing tea. It can be blended with frozen bananas for a fragrant, healthy ice-cream. It is also good for marinating meats and infused into olive oil for a salad dressing.

LIQUORICE is a sweet stick that you can chew on. Real liquorice has a different therapeutic effect from liquorice that is sweetened and bought at candy shops. It has anti-inflammatory, anti-viral and stress relieving properties. It can be used for leaky gut, irritable bowel, crohn's, colitis, bowel spasms, peptic ulcers and mouth ulcers. In Japan it is used for viral hepatitis and in China for tuberculosis.

Tips: It blends well in desserts and makes a delicious tea.

Note: In some people it can cause high blood pressure. If eaten in excess it excretes potassium (which can lead to muscle failure) and is a laxative which may be useful for some.

MINT/PEPPERMINT has a calming, soothing effect on the gut and is cooling. It helps get rid of gas and bloating. It is also helpful if you have nausea or travel sickness and works well with ginger as a tea.

Note: Peppermint tea can reduce iron absorption if taken near a meal (black tea does the same, due to tannins). Avoid if you have salicylate sensitivity or reflux.

Tips: Combine with caraway and fennel for bloating and wind and add with liquorice root for digestive inflammation. The leaves are delicious and refreshing in water with lemon. It can also be used in salads and yoghurt dips. It tastes good in soups and sauces.

OREGANO is a member of the mint family. It has a very high antioxidant score and helps to get rid of fungus in the gut. It contains an antioxidant called carvacrol which is also in thyme, savory, caraway and sweet marjoram. The oil is usually given for fungal (candida) gut problems. It is also effective for giardia and bacteria in the gut. A US study at the Department of Agriculture shows that oregano, rich in cancer fighting quercetin, has the most antioxidant activity of all the herbs. Amazingly it has 42 times more antioxidant activity than apples.

It goes well with fish, salads, tomato dishes and vegetables.

Tips: You can add it to salad dressings and meat dishes with garlic.

PARSLEY is very protective for the immune system and is high in vitamin C. It is also a good cleanser and helps remove fluid from the body. Flat leaf parsley has a stronger flavour than curly parsley and holds up more strongly in cooking.

Tips: It is best to add near the end of cooking to preserve the nutrients. It can garnish any dish and is good in soups and salads. It helps freshen breath and get rid of garlic breath.

ROSEMARY contains a powerful antioxidant, anti-inflammatory (helping peptic ulcers and colitis) and anticancer substance called carnosol. Rosemary is warming and helps improve digestion, circulation and memory. It helps the liver to detoxify and protects the liver from damage. It also helps allergies.

Tips: It seasons roast meats, especially lamb and is good with omelettes, soups and sauces.

SAGE contains antioxidants and phenols including rosmarinic acid which is beneficial for inflammation and is useful in inflammatory bowel disease along with turmeric, basil and liquorice. It's used as a purifying herb.

Note: Sage can stop lactation and is used for menopausal hot flushes.

Tips: It's used in meat stuffing and you can use the leaves as a tea. Chewing on a few leaves is great for bad breath. It was traditionally used as a mouth wash.

STEVIA is a healthy natural sweetener that has a positive effect on the pancreas and helps insulin sensitivity.

TAMARIND helps stomach and liver problems. You can buy the fruit pulp from Asian shops. It has a sour taste and can be added to savoury and sweet dishes or blended with juice.

THYME contains thymol which has many health benefits. It contains flavonoids and carvacrol which help with gastrointestinal problems including diarrhoea, lack of appetite and gut infections. It also protects omega 3 fatty acids in the cells. It benefits the brain and major organs because of its high antioxidant and enzyme activity.

Tips: It combines well with parsley, bay leaves and is good in stocks, stews, soups and sauces. It is also helpful for helicobacter pylori (which causes stomach ulcers).

TURMERIC is a root and looks a bit like ginger but it's yellow or orange. It is also known as curcumin. It's a very powerful anti-inflammatory and will help colic, wind pain, cancer, inflammatory bowel, irritable bowel, especially crohn's and colitis, fissures, peptic ulcers, bowel cancer as well as inflammation caused by parasites.

It also prevents inflammation in the gut lining. Low doses have been shown to be effective for bowel ulceration. It protects the colon from free radicals which can damage DNA. This is very beneficial as colonic cells turn over every three days. Changes in the DNA can form cancer; turmeric helps to stop this and reduces metastasis. It has an amazing ability to help the liver detoxify toxic chemicals by increasing liver enzymes.

Is a powerful antioxidant and helps other antioxidants (like vitamin A, C and E) work better. It reduces the risk of cell damage and slows down the ageing process. It protects bad cholesterol and it helps lower oestrogen. It also lowers blood sugar.

Ideally you need to use heat and oil to extract the active components of turmeric. You can cook it with vegetables in coconut oil or when you are cooking onions and garlic. The fresh root is higher quality than the powder and three tablespoons of fresh root is equivalent to one tablespoon of powder. Turmeric colours everything yellow so make sure you use stainless steel or glass cookware and wear gloves to prevent staining.

To prevent bowel polyps which are a precursor to cancer, cook with the rind of lemons or limes or onions for their quercetin content. A study of five patients with bowel polyps who were given 480 mg curcumin (the active part of turmeric) plus 20 mg quercetin three times a day for six months were shown to decrease their polyps by 60% in volume and 50% in size. Studies have shown that turmeric clears human cancer cells of bowel polyps and cancer.

Note: As an interesting side note, studies have shown that eating foods with turmeric added can reduce the risk of childhood leukaemia. This cancer has risen by 50% in children under 5 since 1950. Environmental and lifestyle factors are thought to play a major role in this increase.

Tips: Chopped with ginger root it works well as an anti-inflammatory tea. It works well in curries, soups and in rice it adds a bright yellow colour. The root is best kept in the fridge but the powder can be kept in a jar like other herbs. Other anti-inflammatory foods include ginger, garlic and liquorice.

Herbal teas

CHAI

5 fresh cloves, 8 cardamom pods, 2 cinnamon sticks, vanilla bean, ¼ whole nutmeg, 8 black peppercorns, 1 tsp. organic green or dandelion tea (optional) chopped ginger.

Slice the vanilla bean, take out the beans and crush in a pestle and mortar. Simmer in 2 cups of filtered water for 10 minutes. Do not boil. Turn the heat off and add other ingredients then let it brew for a minimum of 10 minutes.

Tips: For ease you can make up your own dried mixture and keep it in a glass jar. You can multiply the above mixture as you like. If you want you can add warm rice milk, oat milk, coconut milk or almond milk. This tea aids digestion and helps get rid of mucous and parasites in the body. You don't want to boil the spices as it destroys the aromatic oils. For therapeutic benefits you can drink this on an empty stomach.

CHAMOMILE

This tea helps digestion and is also very calming. As a lot of digestive problems are made worse from worry, this is a lovely tea to have at night and aids a good sleep.

DANDELION ROOT

A good tea for promoting bile from the liver which aids constipation and makes digestion (particularly fats) easier.

FLAXSEED TEA

It is very good for healing the intestines especially if you have leaky gut, irritable bowel syndrome, spasm type pain in the gut, inflammatory bowel disease or blood in your stools.

Pour boiling water over a tablespoon of whole flaxseeds into a large mug and leave for at least half an hour or overnight if possible. Drain and drink the liquid daily.

GREEN TEA

This tea has just enough caffeine to pick you up but is much lower in caffeine than black tea and coffee so is less irritating to the gut and a better alternative if you have not yet come off caffeine. It is packed with powerful antioxidants which have many health benefits.

Tips: If you add milk to green tea it completely stops the antioxidant activity. Regular tea affects the nervous and digestive system with 3 stimulants; caffeine, theophylline and theobromine. Caffeine is highest in coffee, theophylline in tea and theobromine in chocolate.

KUKICHA

This is a Japanese twig tea and is very low in caffeine. It alkalises the digestive system, settles the stomach and helps detoxify the body.

LEMONGRASS AND GINGER

Mix chopped ginger and chopped lemongrass stick for a refreshing digestive tea.

LEMON VERBENA

This is very easy to grow in a pot in your garden. I love this tea and have been growing it for years. It has a lovely lemon aroma. Put 5-10 leaves in a plunger with hot water and let it sit for 5-10 minutes. This is a great digestive and is also calming and restoring to the nervous system.

LIQUORICE (see herbs)

MEADOWSWEET TEA is a superior digestive remedy and protects and soothes mucous membranes in the gut. It blends well with liquorice.

NETTLE

The main use of this herb/tea/leaf is as a cleansing and detoxifying agent in the body. Detoxification of the body is an important property of nettles. Nettle helps cleanse the body of all accumulated toxins and in the rapid removal of metabolic waste.

It alleviates fluid retention. It is used in the treatment of various bladder infections and in the destruction of stones and gravel in the body. It is effective in aiding in the excretion of accumulated uric acid.

Bleeding in any area of the body is treatable by the strong astringent action so it is useful for colitis where bleeding can occur. It can be used in cases of haemorrhoids. It is high in iron and minerals.

PEPPERMINT

A great digestive tea that aids nausea.

SPICE MIX

Mix 4 cloves, 2cm chopped ginger, 4 cardamom pods, ½ teaspoon of fennel seeds and a teaspoon of lemon peel. Heat slowly and have a glass a night for at least a month to improve your digestion.

MUCOUS RELIEVING TEA

If you have a thick coating on your tongue, have over-consumed dairy, wheat, sugar, eggs or meat, or have a snotty nose, this tea will help you.

Mix in a glass jar: 1 tsp. fennel, 1 tsp. fenugreek, 1 tsp. flaxseeds, 1 tsp. nettle leaf, ½ tsp. liquorice root. Drink 1-2 cups a day for at least 4 weeks.

CHAPTER 12

Amazingly Healthy Recipes

*"Now, good digestion wait on appetite,
and health on both."*

Shakespeare

CHAPTER 12
Amazingly Healthy Recipes

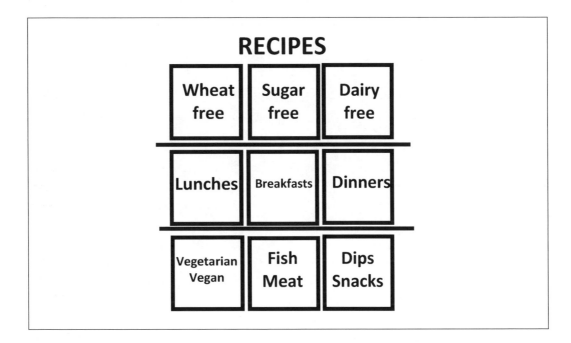

Over the next few pages you will find simply delicious healthy recipes that are easy to make and will greatly improve your digestion.

Eating only one way negates the principles of Chinese and Ayurvedic medicine. These traditional medicines diagnose people in different ways e.g. cold, damp, hot and dry. All foods have these qualities and correspond to individual diagnosis. Someone who is cold and damp would need to avoid dairy, wheat and sugar. Food also affects your personality, for example, someone who has a bright red tongue and is overheated may become angry and irritable if they eat too much meat, chillies and curries whereas this may suit a person who is lethargic, cold and with little energy.

Cooked or raw?

There are some fad diets out there and as everyone is different no diet suits all people. For example, some people thrive on a raw food diet while others find it difficult. If you have a strong digestion raw food may be beneficial. Whilst raw food contains more minerals, enzymes and vitamins, a person needs to be able to digest them. Often those with a damaged gut need to start with soups and easily digested foods.

Some people with certain constitutions and weak digestion cannot handle raw food easily especially if they feel the cold or have had chronic gut problems. We are drawn to the cooling properties of raw foods in summer but in cool climates over consumption of raw foods can cause imbalances in our bodies.

As digestion is essential for health it is wise to have soups, stews, (cooked at low temperatures to preserve nutrients) fermented foods, digestive herbs, warm foods, and drinks so that nutrients can be easily assimilated. Over eating raw or cold foods can slow down digestion. It is important that your body can assimilate what you eat.

Think of your digestion like a pot of soup over a gas flame. The flame is your digestive fire which relies on the function of your stomach, pancreas and liver (the burner). The food in the pot is the food you eat. The burner controls the flame to transform the food so that good nutrition can be absorbed by your body. If you add junk food, cold food or too much raw food it requires more work from the burner to turn up the flame. Over time the burner can weaken causing undigested stools, bloating, gas and other symptoms.

Over eating excess fried, fatty and spicy foods can cause excess heat which leads to toxicity and inflammation. The amount of cold to warm foods needs to suit a person's system to achieve good health.

Fruit is not beneficial for candida, parasites and bloating except for lemons and limes. A lot of people with digestive problems lack digestive energy and fruit weakens this further. Each person's case is individual but often fruit is over consumed and not enough vegetables are eaten.

Having said that, most people do well with a salad before each meal as it stimulates their digestion in a positive way. Fermented vegetables are easy to digest and a small amount at each meal often really helps the digestion.

Cooking food

As you cook, be aware of what you need to do to get the maximum nutrition from your food. This includes avoiding processed and denatured foods. Feel what is good for you. Different cultures see the cook as having a profound effect on the food they prepare, to give a physiological, mental and emotional effect on the body.

It is important to only use coconut oil, rice bran oil, ghee or butter as cooking fats. Damaged fats, additives, contaminants and preservatives all have a negative effect on the body.

Blessing food according to your beliefs has an effect on the vibration of food. In a study, two groups of non-organic food were both prayed over or blessed with Reiki; both were shown to elevate their vibrations, similar to organic food; this was found with Kirlian photography.

Shopping for food

You may have a lifestyle where you go out for dinner often or get take-away after a long day. One in 30 Australians have purchased pre-prepared meals at some time and it's growing. It provides a solution for busy people and it is estimated that 70% of mothers work outside the home yet still do most of the shopping, cooking and meal planning. There are ways to eat healthy meals within your busy life. Planning your meals is very important to keep you eating healthy foods even at busy times. Buying a crock pot can make life easier and so does freezing food.

The ingredients for the recipes ideally need to be organic or at least pesticide free e.g. from farmers markets. It is important to wash all your vegetables in a safe veggie wash (from the health shop). You can buy washing bowls from the $2 shop. Place your vegetables and fruit in the bowl, add (preferably filtered) water, add a few drops of veggie wash and let it sit for 5 minutes. Rinse thoroughly in a colander. If you do this after you shop you can then store already washed produce in the fridge, saving time later.

As a food wash or disinfectant you can also add 1-4 drops of iodine to 1 litre of water and soak your vegetables and fruit for 3-5 minutes then rinse as above. Even if vegetables and fruits are organic they still need to be washed well to get rid of bugs and possible parasite eggs. If you have gut problems you need to be more mindful about washing food as you are more sensitive to picking up these bugs. If you have been very ill I would suggest cooking all your vegetables at a low heat and avoiding fruit. Iodine is also useful to take when travelling in order to wash food.

To clean surfaces in the kitchen I use 50% apple cider vinegar with water to spray my cutting board, sink and counter instead of bleach.

Recipes

All the recipes are wheat free, mostly gluten free, dairy free, sugar free and use only natural ingredients. They cater for most digestive problems however, some people who don't respond to these kind of foods and have tried everything may have to go on a stricter diet.

For those people, I highly recommend the specific carbohydrate diet (SCD) and the elemental diet for a minimum of six weeks. It requires a lot of dedication to do it, but it makes such a huge difference that you will be encouraged to keep going. I have found that some people on the SCD cannot handle all the nuts (they need liver work) and for some I have added chia seeds and ground linseeds to give more fibre if they are constipated.

You will notice that some of the following recipes are raw. Cooked recipes are best cooked slowly to avoid nutrient loss; at around 100 degrees in a slow cooker. The recipes contain extraordinary health and gut benefits and taste superb. There are also specific recipes in the chapters on ferments and kitchen pharmacy.

Some of the recipes, especially the dips, have yoghurt. This is very therapeutic in small amounts and organic yoghurt is the only one to use. You can use kefir if you want an abundance of probiotics. About two tablespoons of yoghurt twice a day is recommended for health benefits. Over indulgence in yoghurt causes congestion in the body. The lymphatics congest, the intestines congest and mucous forms, which is a breeding ground for bacteria. It needs to be decreased in cold, damp weather or if you are cold and have a coating on your tongue. It is best not eaten in the evening when the digestion is weaker.

All nuts in the recipes are best activated. To do this you can buy them activated or soak them for at least 4 hours then eat them. If you want to keep them, drain off the water and dry them in a very low oven for about 8 hrs until they are dry, then store in a glass jar in the fridge.

It's time to start cooking. Cooking is an adventure and by understanding why various ingredients are used, how they affect the body or what purpose they serve in a dish, leads to a satisfying experience not a tiresome chore.

Recipes

10 tips for enjoying cooking

1. Organise your kitchen with the utensils you need and have them near the work bench and stove.

2. Have good quality cookware and a blender. If you want high quality and versatility I recommend Vitamix (www.vitamix.com.au). I'd also recommend a juicer. You can get juicers that don't use blades to destroy nutrients like a compact juicer does and there are various high end juicers on the market.

3. Have good quality knives and cutting boards, scales, garlic press, scissors and a good stock of herbs spices and quality oils.

4. Organise your week and plan ahead so you can buy everything you need to make your cooking experience easier.

5. Take deep breaths and get yourself relaxed. Get yourself in a good mood; if you need music or aromatherapy oils to enhance your experience, use them. Your vibration affects your food. Avoid tasting the food and putting the same utensil back into the food. Enzymes from saliva may cause spoilage, cross contaminate and change the vibration of the food. Of course taste it, but wash the spoon if you taste it again.

6. Have respect and gratitude for the food you are going to eat. Think about all the processes and people needed to grow the food and get it to you. This is also likely to get you eating healthy food!

7. Organise the time you will need. You may need to soak things the night before or you may put the slow cooker on before you go to work for a yummy meal in the evening.

8. As you get used to cooking, use your intuition and creativity to select colour, taste, shapes and smells. I do this all the time and I wouldn't be without fresh herbs to add flavour to cooked foods and salads. I usually have pots of basil, oregano, parsley and coriander growing outside the kitchen. Get to know the healing effects of food (for example turmeric is fantastic for bowel inflammation) and bring out the tastes and flavours. You can preserve the life force by cooking at low temperatures and having raw food if you can digest it.

9. Keep it simple, until you are familiar with cooking and making easy healthy recipes, avoid complicated recipes unless you are experienced. Allow time to clean and if you clean up as you go, it will leave a lot less mess afterwards.

10. Set the scene. If it's only you, make sure you sit down; you can light a candle or put a flower on the table and use utensils you enjoy, making it a mindful and pleasant experience. Avoid putting the best things away for special guests; treat yourself like a special guest. Make the effort to cook for someone you love or someone who inspires you.

A message from Kiran who has contributed some Indian dishes:

"For me, the secret of cooking good food is very simple, use good ingredients, give thanks for the food and more importantly cook with love. There is nothing quite like eating food that has been lovingly prepared and cooked; it just tastes better! Try and you'll see. I have always believed that the energy we carry when doing anything affects the outcome and cooking is no different. I have a rule that if I'm not feeling in a good mood I will not cook because I don't want to pass my negative energy onto anyone. Cooking with love is the key ingredient in all my dishes and I hope it will be in yours too."

Special appliances

High powered blenders Vitamix

www.vitamix.com

Powerful Food processors

www.kitchen-universe.com

www.robotcoupeusa.com

Recipes

The recipes serve about 4 people depending on their appetite, unless otherwise stated.

7 wheat free, dairy free, sugar free breakfasts that taste delicious

These recipes are for 1 or 2 people

1. **OATBRAN CEREAL -** add boiling water to ½ cup of oat bran, mix until it becomes like porridge. You can add chia seeds, L.S.A. (ground linseeds, sunflower seeds and almonds), berries and two figs. Add rice milk or coconut milk and flaxseed oil as you like.

Tips: This is a very high fibre breakfast and oat bran on its own is a quick and easy breakfast. You can add ginger for easier digestion. You can use any of these fibres in the other breakfasts.

2. **BUCKWHEAT PANCAKES -** Mix 1 cup of buckwheat or another flour of your choice, 1 beaten egg, some water or rice milk to get the consistency you want. Some people like thin pancakes, some like them thick. Place into a shallow frying pan with some coconut oil, cook and turn when brown. Spread a healthy dip on it or berries and yoghurt. For those with a sweet tooth you can add 2 tbsp. of carob powder and desiccated coconut to the mix. For a coffee flavour, add chicory powder. You can add a variety of dressings, mashed avocado, tomatoes, buffalo cheese, rice syrup, sliced banana, coconut milk or oil.

Tips: Add one teaspoon of cinnamon powder; you can also use oat milk or almond milk or coconut milk. Use topping ideas above. It's great for Sunday brunch. Those who can't tolerate any flours can use almond meal instead. Buckwheat is good for haemorrhoids. You can also make it with rye flour; as it is heavy; adding tapioca flour makes it more digestible.

3. **BROWN RICE CEREAL** you can use brown rice, quinoa or buckwheat cooked the night before. Heat the grain. If you prefer you can heat it until it becomes like a porridge (congee). Once cooked add sunflower seeds, pumpkins seeds, a teaspoon of bee pollen, kefir or yoghurt or a milk of your choice.

Tips: If you want it savoury crack a couple of eggs on it and then add sesame seeds, tamari and avocado.

4. **TASTY OMELETTE** - beat two eggs and add tsp. of chopped shallots, ½ tsp. coriander, ½ tsp. mint leaves, ¼ cup chopped red capsicum, ½ cup chopped parsley and a pinch of Celtic salt.

Tips: You can add this to brown rice, or sweet potato and tamari. Always add something green to eggs to help balance the acid with alkaline.

5. **FISH SURPRISE** on a buckwheat pancake - add chopped tomatoes, avocado and sardines with cracked pepper and olive oil.

Tips: You can vary the veg with rocket, spinach or alfalfa sprouts.

6. **SPICED MILLET -** this is high in protein and fibre. You can add a grain if you wish. Put a few tbsp. of millet in a bowl with a large sprinkling of sesame seeds and a smaller sprinkling of fennel seeds, add a little olive oil and water, mix and fry in coconut oil until crisp.

Tips: You can add fennel seeds, which have a wonderful distinct Indian flavour, to any of the recipes for easier digestion. Also add your quantity of sunflower, pumpkin and fennel seeds, sesame seeds, linseeds and cinnamon to a bowl and soak overnight in yoghurt or milk.

7. **POLENTA PORRIDGE** - heat 2 cups of goat's or sheep's milk or a milk of your choice, add 4 tbsp. maize flour and a little sago flour stirring all the time until you reach the desired consistency. Top with pecans or walnuts.

Tips: Add ginger and fennel seeds for easier digestion. A great warming winter breakfast and also good as a snack or dessert (cinnamon and coconut cream are good in a dessert).

DIGESTIVE DRINKS

Start the day with fresh filtered water and half a lemon or lime. For a bit more taste, add some mint leaves. This is lovely to serve guests.

ATTRACTIVE ICE CUBES

You can also add ice cubes with edible flowers. Make sure the flowers are organically grown.

¼ fill the ice tray with water. Add the flowers face down then top up with water and freeze. These look beautiful. As an example, you can add nasturtiums, borage, marigold, hibiscus or chamomile. These are a delightful way to serve a drink on a hot summer's day. Remember to avoid the habit of ice cubes, as warm water is better for the digestion.

TUMMY COMFORT

1 tsp. chopped fresh ginger
Small bunch of mint leaves
½ tsp. bicarb. soda
½ lemon
1 litre of water

Method:

Blend all ingredients.

Tip: For severe indigestion have ½ tsp. bicarb only in water before bed. Buy organic bicarb from a health shop.

METABOLISER

This is a powerful drink and a great way to help weight loss; drink it in the morning.

Blend:

½ tsp. cayenne pepper
Juice of 1 lemon
Water as desired
Pineapple or kiwi as desired

GALL BLADDER LIVER DRINK

This drink is strong and excellent for stimulating bile to help your liver and gall bladder.

½ tsp. cayenne
1 clove garlic
2 tbsp. olive oil
Juice of 1 lemon
Water as desired
Optional: pinch of turmeric and tomato juice

Blend all ingredients.

LIMEADE

The juice of 1 lime with 200mls of sparkling mineral water and a sprinkling of cinnamon.

Tip: Mint is optional.

SOOTHING LASSI MAKES 2 REFRESHING DRINKS

1 tall glass of kefir or yoghurt
½-1 orange papaya depending on size
½ tsp. ginger

A few mint leaves
2 pitted prunes or figs

Blend together

Tips: You can add a sprinkling of cinnamon to the top of the glass if you like.

GINGER TEA

Juice 4 tbsp. of ginger and add warm water for a soothing digestive tea.

SPICE DIGESTIVE TEA

Cloves
Cinnamon
Ginger
Nutmeg

Tips: To help your liver and constipation mix this with dandelion root. This tea is also good to take for 8 weeks (2 cups a day) to help get rid of parasite eggs.

Vegetable juices serve 1

These are best with half water to slow the absorption of natural sugars.

MORNING ZINGER

In a juicer combine:

1 cucumber
6 sticks of celery
½ bunch parsley
1 tomato optional
Lemon optional
Small pinch of chilli or cayenne pepper

RED BOOSTER - BY GRACE

Ingredients: Add the quantities you desire

Beetroot (good for iron)
Celery
Garlic, peeled - very good for parasites and antiseptic to the bowel.

Method:

Juice beetroot and celery. Blend with garlic and water. You can serve with ice.

Tip: Garlic is quite strong but the celery will balance the strong flavour of garlic. You may only need 1-2 cloves of garlic for 1 drink of 360-400ml.

DRINK YOUR GREENS - BY GRACE

Ingredients: Choose your own quantities

Spinach and/or kale
Pineapple - once you can tolerate fruit, pineapple contains bromelain which helpsdigestion

Method:

Blend spinach and kale with a small piece of pineapple and water. Add water if necessary.

Tip: For faster bowel movement, adding a fig is recommended.

POWERFUL GREEN DELIGHT

Ingredients: ¼ cucumber

I handful coriander leaves
1 handful parsley
2 inches chopped ginger

½ peeled lemon
Juice the above ingredients
1-2 cups of coconut water

Method:

Add the juice to the coconut water

DIGESTIVE POWER

½ cup of kefir or yoghurt and 1 cup water, 4 cardamom pods, 1 tsp. of cinnamon and fennel as desired. Whiz it up in a food processor. It is also nice with fennel seeds. You can alter ingredients as desired. For a more sustaining drink add half an avocado.

MILK SPICE

Use nut milks or rice or almond milk and add a few cardamom pods, heat and serve warm with a sprinkling of cinnamon.

I rarely recommend fruit juices however, if you are well on the mend an occasional fresh juice or smoothie may sit well. If you have any bloating or discomfort, stick with lemon, water and vegetable juices.

Smoothies

TROPICAL ENZYME SMOOTHIE

1 cup coconut water
1 cup pineapple (bromelain helps digestion)
1 cup chopped pawpaw
Pinch sea salt

Variation: 1 cup coconut water, 1 date, tsp. turmeric (soaked in a small amount of hot water for 2 minutes for inflammation), 1tsp ginger, 1 tsp. cardamom

MIXED DELIGHT

1 avocado

1tsp. carob powder

½ tsp. stevia

5 kale leaves

1 cup organic yoghurt or kefir

1 tsp vanilla extract

¼ cup raw tahini

2 tablespoons chia seeds

Small handful pecan nuts

1 cup filtered water

Method:

Blend all ingredients and add more water if necessary. For variations add cinnamon, carob, figs for fibre, berries, or mint.

7 mouth-watering soups

1.   RED PEPPER SOUP

Ingredients:

1 cup coconut water or filtered water

½ cup of blended macadamia nuts

2 cups of chopped red capsicum

½ tsp. Celtic sea salt

½ tsp. rice syrup or yacon syrup or honey

½ tsp. paprika powder

1 tsp. coconut oil

Pinch cayenne pepper

Method:

Blend all ingredients in a high powered blender until smooth. This can be eaten cold or warm.

Tip: Blended food is great for the tummy as it does not require extra energy for breaking down the food. You can blend all the soups if you need to.

2. RECOVERY RICE SOUP

If your tummy is feeling weak or you have vomited and you are recovering this is a good way to start on food.

Ingredients:

Arborio rice, white short grain or basmati rice

Method:

Boil the rice in 5 times the water for 45 minutes. Add a pinch of Celtic salt and a teaspoon of coconut oil.

Tip: If your digestion is poor you can just take the liquid off the soup. You can also blend it with a little ginger.

3. MISO TUMMY SOUP

Ingredients:

1 onion finely chopped
3 cm fresh ginger grated
3 cloves garlic finely chopped
Small bunch of coriander; finely chop the leaves and the roots
1 large carrot chopped
1 daikon radish chopped (great for the liver)
1 cup of pumpkin cubed

2 handfuls of green beans chopped

1 head of broccoli chopped

½ bunch of Asian greens chopped

4 shitake mushrooms, soaked in warm water for 15 minutes then chopped

1 strip Wakame seaweed, rinsed and cut into thin strips with scissors then soaked in warm water for 15 minutes

A handful of Arame seaweed, soaked in warm water for 15 minutes

1 packet silken tofu, cubed

4 heaped teaspoons of miso dissolved in a cup of water

8 cups of water

2 tbsp. rice bran oil or coconut oil

Shallots, finely chopped for garnish

Method:

Heat the oil in a large saucepan and gently sauté the onions for a few minutes, then add the garlic, ginger and coriander roots. Stir in the carrots, pumpkin and daikon radish until sweaty then add the water, bring to almost boiling then simmer for 15 minutes. Add the beans, tofu and shitake and all the greens, simmer for 15 minutes. Turn off the heat and add dissolved miso. Garnish with shallots.

Tip: This serves 4-6 people. You can make up large batches and freeze it. It is a very nutritious soup that you can take out of the freezer on busy days. It is antiseptic, warming and soothing for the gut. It is packed with vitamins, minerals and probiotics and the shitake mushrooms do wonders for the immune system. If you have candida and are sensitive to miso just leave it out and use herb salt.

You can vary the types of vegetables you use. For less preparation use nori seaweed or dulse which doesn't require soaking. It is delicious served with brown rice or over soba noodles. You can buy soba noodles from a health shop and make sure you get ones that are 100% buckwheat with no added wheat. Cook as directed on the packet.

A word on tofu:

It is fine to use occasionally but I would always cook it with warming herbs and spices as it is very cooling. In China they put strips of it on children's foreheads to cool them down when they have a fever. Never use raw, it puts too much stress on your digestion. I have seen dessert recipes with raw tofu and I don't recommend it.

4.   KNOCK OUT PARASITE BORSCHT SOUP

Ingredients:

6 beetroots sliced
1 carrot sliced
1 small red cabbage sliced
1 sweet potato sliced
1 onion diced
1 lemon juiced
Coconut oil
1 clove garlic diced
4 cloves (place in a tea strainer or muslin cloth and remove after cooking)
Stock to taste
Pinch black pepper
Pinch fennel
Pinch thyme
Pinch oregano
1 tbsp. chopped parsley

Method:

Sauté onion and garlic for 2 minutes then add herbs and a litre of water. Add other ingredients and cook for 30 minutes. Blend. Add lemon juice and parsley at the end.

5. GREEN CURRIED AVOCADO SOUP- BY GRACE

Ingredients for 1 serve of 400ml:

1 avocado
Handful of spinach (baby spinach is great)
Pinch of Himalayan salt
Pinch of coriander seeds
Pinch of cumin seeds
Pinch of pepper (preferably raw)
Water (as much as you like to get a smooth consistency but not too thick)
Pinch of fresh chilli (optional)
Coriander leaves and/or alfalfa sprouts

Method:

Blend all ingredients. Garnish with fresh cilantro or alfalfa sprouts and sprinkle with nigella seeds or sesame seeds. Add turmeric for an anti-inflammatory effect. Add a tsp. of whole flaxseeds for a soothing effect.

Variations

IRON BOOSTER SOUP:

Celery
Mushrooms
Parsley stalks
Garnish with fresh parsley leaves
Beetroot

Cheesy avocado soup:
A bit more spinach
Yeast flakes (not for candida)
Garnish with fresh dill

6. THAI GREEN SOUP: BY GRACE

Galanghal (or ginger)
Lemon grass
Kaffir lime leaves
Green chilli
Sprouted beans (not blended, just added to the soup)
Garnish with Vietnamese mint

Tip: If you haven't got any seeds (cumin/coriander) available, use curry powder instead. It will not be the same fresh taste but will do the job! Go Mexican with some fresh corn added, red chilli and spouted beans. Have fun and positive thoughts while chopping, blending, mixing and eating!

7. PUMPKIN SOUP WITH TURMERIC AND GINGER BY GRACE

Ingredients: Choose your ingredient amounts

Pumpkin, peeled and chopped into small cubes
Turmeric, preferably fresh, if not available, dry powder will do
Ginger, freshly grated
Coriander seeds
Olive oil or rice bran oil
Cinnamon, ground
Nutmeg, ground
Stock or water
Salt, pepper, chilli

Method:

Heat the oil in a pan. Sautee ginger, turmeric and coriander seeds. Once you can smell the flavour, add pumpkin and fry together. Add nutmeg and cinnamon and fry for just a little longer stirring continuously now to prevent burning. Add water or stock and bring to the boil. Once boiling, turn the heat down and simmer. Blend the soup and season per your preference with salt, cinnamon and pepper.

Tip: Add chilli if you like spicy food. With spices, start small with 1 tbsp. of coriander seeds and after you make it once, you will know how you like it best. Next time add less or more. Do the same with cinnamon and nutmeg; use as much or as little as you like.

A ginger flavour will come up better if you grate half of the ginger for frying and blend the other half with water or stock and add it at the end of cooking.

6 Healthy Dips

Dips make good snacks and they can also be used to dress food, not only salads but also meat, fish and legume dishes.

1.   TOMATO SPICE

Add one tin of organic tomatoes with one avocado, blend with juice of half a lemon, a little salt and coriander.

Tip: You can vary herbs and spices to taste. If you like spice add I tsp. curry powder. Also good for toddlers.

2.   QUICK CHICKPEA DIP

Ingredients:

I tin of organic chick peas
4 tbs. virgin olive oil
2 cloves garlic
½ tsp. cumin
Pinch chilli flakes (optional)
Juice ½ lemon
Handful parsley
1 tbsp. tahini (optional)
½ tsp. fine Celtic salt

Put everything in a blender until creamy. If it is too thick add more oil, some water or lemon juice and taste for seasoning. Easy and delicious.

Tip: For economy, buy organic dried chick peas and soak them overnight.

3. YOGHURT AND CUCUMBER DIP

Ingredients:

1 cup of organic plain yoghurt
1 cucumber peeled and chopped
1 tablespoon of apple cider vinegar
1 tbsp. crushed dill
¼ tsp. powdered cumin seeds
¼ tsp. black pepper
1 tbsp. chopped coriander
1 clove garlic chopped finely
1 tsp. chopped mint.

Method:

Dry roast the cumin seeds and crush to a powder. Blend all ingredients.

Tip: For something different, add chopped walnuts or pecans. This is very good for your digestion; if you are sensitive to garlic, leave it out.

4. GINGER ZEST DIP

Ingredients:

1 cup of almond meal or plain yoghurt
Juice of 1 lemon
1 tbsp. grated lemon rind (make sure it's organic)
1 tbsp. grated ginger

1 clove garlic crushed

1 tbsp. apple cider vinegar

Method:

Blend all ingredients in a food processor.

Tip: If you use almond meal add some water for desired consistency.

5. PURPLE CLEANSER DIP

Ingredients:

1 average sized beetroot

1 cup toasted pumpkin seeds or sunflowers seeds

A pinch of cayenne pepper

1 tsp. mustard seeds

Juice of 2 lemons

½ cup water

½ tsp. Celtic or Himalayan salt

Method:

Blend all ingredients in a food processor.

Tip: If you don't have seeds, use nuts. This is high in zinc which heals the bowel. It is also high in iron and vitamin C for healing and alkaline which will benefit your gut.

6. MINT AND GINGER DIP

Ingredients:

60 g fresh mint or coriander leaves

¼ tsp. black pepper

1 tbsp. grated ginger

3 tbsp. of lime or lemon juice

½ tsp. of Celtic or Himalayan salt

Method:

Blend all ingredients in a food processor until smooth.

Tip: This is wonderful for your digestion. Add a little olive oil in the blender. If you are sensitive to pepper leave it out.

7 Scrumptious salads

1.   WALNUT SALAD

Ingredients:

2 cups of shredded beetroot

2 cloves chopped garlic

½ cup chopped walnuts

Pinch celtic sea salt

Mix together

Dressing:

½ cup pine nuts

½ cup cashew nuts (soaked for two hours)

1 tbsp. lime or lemon juice

1 tsp. sea salt

1 tsp. rice syrup

½ cup chopped radish

¼ cup purified water

½ tsp. chopped ginger

2 tbsp. chopped red onion

Method:

Blend in a food processor or with a bar mixer until smooth then toss it through the salad.

Tip: Beetroot contains nitric oxide which has amazing health benefits for stamina. Adding a bunch of rocket and goat's cheese works well.

2.   BEETROOT SALAD

Ingredients:

1 large beetroot
1 large grated carrot
4 tbsp. desiccated coconut or sesame seeds

Dressing:

The juice of 1 orange, lime or lemon and 2 tbsp. olive oil or rice bran oil

Method:

Combine all ingredients and serve with a meal.

Tip: Beetroot is a great cleanser for the gut. It is high in iron and vitamin C and easy to absorb.

3.   BEAN SPROUT SALAD

Ingredients:

3 cups bean sprouts
1 cup grated carrots
1 green pepper sliced finely

Dressing:

1 tbsp. olive oil, 1 tbsp. sesame oil, 1 tbsp. tamari, 2 tbsp. apple cider vinegar

Method:

Combine all ingredients and serve with a meal.

4. WAKAME AND CUCUMBER SALAD

Ingredients:

30 grams Wakame soaked for 15 minutes then drained and chopped
1 cucumber sliced
5 radishes thinly sliced
2 tbsp. lemon juice
1 tbsp. shoyu
1 tbsp. spring onions to garnish

Method:

Combine all ingredients and serve with a meal.

5. MUNG BEAN SALAD

Ingredients:

1 cup dried mung beans soaked overnight and cooked for 20 minutes
½ cup cooked brown rice
¼ cup almonds
2 tbsp. tahini
¼ cup chopped parsley, onion and chives
2 cloves chopped garlic
Blend above ingredients (which can also be used for a dip) then add
½ cup Bok choy chopped and ½ cup celery chopped.

6.   GREEN SALAD

Ingredients:

½ cup chopped bok choy
½ cup chopped lettuce
A handful of grilled sunflower and pumpkin seeds (until they go brown)
200g soaked Wakame
2 chopped shallots
¼ cup apple cider vinegar
¼ cup olive oil

Blend together.

7.   LAZY SUNDAY SALAD

Ingredients:

Large handful rocket

Large handful alfalfa sprouts
Large handful chopped parsley
Sprinkle of sunflower and sesame seeds
½ juice lemon
Olive oil to taste and garlic if desired

Method: Blend all ingredients. It goes well with eggs or goat's cheese.

13   Delicious mains - meat/fish/vegan/vegetarian

1.   LAMB MEATBALLS WITH GREEN CURRY SAUCE

This is delicious served top of brown rice or buckwheat noodles.

Ingredients:

For the meatballs:
1 pound or 2 cups of minced lamb
1 tsp. grated fresh ginger root
1 tbsp. chopped Thai or cinnamon basil
1 tbsp. chopped coriander leaves
½ tsp. ground cumin
½ tsp. ground coriander
1 egg - beaten
¼ cup chia seeds

Method:

Preheat your oven to 350°F. In a large bowl add all the ingredients and mix well. Using a tbsp. form the mixture into meatballs. Place the meatballs onto a baking tray and bake in the oven for 20 minutes. Makes approximately 30 meatballs. While the meatballs are cooking you can prepare the sauce.

GREEN CURRY SAUCE

Ingredients:

2 tbsp. coconut oil
2 cups chopped leeks
2 cups sliced mushrooms
½ tsp. ground cumin
½ tsp. ground coriander

1 tsp. Celtic salt

1 tbsp. thinly sliced fresh kaffir lime leaves

1 tsp. grated fresh ginger root

2 tsp. thinly sliced fresh curry leaves

1 tbsp. chopped hot chilli pepper

1 can unsweetened coconut milk (available from health shops)

½ cup water

Method:

Add the coconut oil to a saucepan and place it over medium heat. Add the leeks and cook for 5 minutes. Add the mushrooms, cumin, coriander and salt and cook for another 4 minutes. Add the kaffir lime leaves, ginger root, curry leaves and chilli pepper and cook for 1 more minute. Add the coconut milk and water and stir well. Cook for another two minutes until the sauce is bubbly. When the meatballs are done, place them in a large bowl and pour the sauce over them. Makes 5 servings of approximately 6 meatballs per serving.

2.   KAFFIR LIME CHILLI

This is delicious served over brown rice or quinoa. This dish can also be used on burritos if desired. It can be used as a dip with organic blue corn chips. You can make this dish as a dip adding ¼ cup olive oil.

Ingredients:

1 cup diced onions

1 pound or 2 cups minced lamb, kangaroo or beef or chickpeas or tofu

4 cloves minced garlic

2 cans organic diced tomatoes or cooked fresh tomatoes

¼ tsp. chilli powder

1 tsp. turmeric

½ tsp. salt - optional

½ tsp. black pepper

1 can organic black beans or cooked dried beans

1 can whole organic kernel corn or 2 cooked corn (remove kernels)

1 tbsp. fresh kaffir lime leaves - sliced thin

1 tbsp. minced fresh oregano

1 tbsp. minced fresh marjoram

1 tbsp. fresh lemon thyme leaves

Juice and zest from 1 lime

Method:

Add coconut oil to a large saucepan over a medium heat, stir in the onions and cook for 5 minutes. Add the minced meat and cook for 5 more minutes. Stir in the garlic and cook for 1 more minute. Stir in the tomatoes, chilli, salt, black pepper and simmer over medium low heat for 10 minutes. Stir in black beans, corn, kaffir lime leaves, turmeric, oregano, marjoram and thyme and simmer for an additional 20 minutes. Remove the pan from the heat and stir in the lime juice and lime zest and serve immediately. Makes approximately 8-10 servings.

3. **DISH TO REDUCE BLOOD SUGAR AND INFLAMMATION**

Ingredients:

1 chopped bitter melon

1 cup diced beef or other meat or chickpeas

1 chopped onion

2 cloves garlic

1 tsp. chopped turmeric

1 tsp. chopped ginger

Handful coriander

1 chopped zucchini

1 chopped carrot

1 bunch bok choy

1 red capsicum

Coconut oil

Salt to taste

Method:

Put the onion, garlic, turmeric, ginger and carrot in a frying pan with olive oil and beef. Whilst that is cooking cut the bitter melon in half and scoop out the seeds, then chop into 1 inch size pieces and put in a pan with boiling salted water for 2-4 minutes. Then drain the water and add the bitter melon to the frying pan. Add zucchini and put a lid on the pan for 3 minutes. Then add bok choy and coriander for about 2 minutes putting back the lid. Serve with a handful of raw capsicum on top.

4.   CHICKEN CURRY BY KIRAN

Serves 4

Ingredients:

1 tbsp. rice bran oil
1 tsp. of cumin seeds
3 medium organic onions diced roughly
3 cloves of organic garlic diced roughly
400g of diced organic tomatoes
3cm cube of organic ginger quartered
2 Birdseye chillies (more if you prefer it hot)
Salt to taste
1 tsp. turmeric powder
Handful of baby spinach
600g free range chicken thigh fillets, fat trimmed and cut into 2 inch cubes
2-3 tsp. garam masala
Jug of water
Small handful of fresh chopped coriander to garnish

Method:

Heat the oil in a large cooking pot with lid, add the cumin seeds and cook on a medium heat for 2 minutes, releasing the flavour. Add the onions and garlic and cook on medium to high heat until onions are browned (approx. 15 mins). Add a little water if onions are sticking to the pot and stir the onions often.

Place the chillies and ginger in a mini food processor and blitz. Add this mixture and the tomatoes to the onions and then add the turmeric and salt and cook for 5-8 minutes. (Note: add a little water if mixture looks too dry).

Add the spinach, then turn the gas to low and stir, cooking for a further 5 minutes. Turn the gas off and using the pureeing attachment on your blender, puree the mixture in the pot. (Note: if using a non-stick pot for cooking ensure that you first empty the mixture in a large glass bowl prior to pureeing and return to pot afterwards). Puree on medium speed, adding water to make the sauce the consistency you prefer. Once this is done turn the gas to medium.

Add the chicken and garam masala to the sauce and cook for approx. 12 minutes on a medium to high heat or until chicken is cooked, ensuring you stir often.

Once cooked add the chopped coriander and serve with basmati rice or roti (Indian flat bread).

5. EASY FISH DISH

Please note: Eat low mercury fish.

Avoid sword fish, marlin, shark/flake, orange roughy/deep sea perch and catfish.

Limit: Barramundi, gemfish, ling, tuna, halibut, mahimahi, sea bass.

Choose fish of your choice. Very good with salmon.

Ingredients:

Sauce

Bunch of coriander
Bunch of shallots finely chopped
Tsp of ginger finely chopped

2 Garlic cloves finely chopped

Juice of one lime and a tablespoon of lime zest.

Method:

Mix sauce ingredients and spoon over fish. Bake at 180°C for 15 minutes.

Tips: Goes well with quinoa.

6.   FISH CAKES

Ingredients:

400 g sweet potatoes, scrubbed

400 g cauliflower, trimmed and cut into florets

300 g wild salmon quickly poached.

1 red chilli, chopped finely

½ teaspoon lemon rind

1 tablespoon lemon juice

3 shallots, finely sliced

2 tablespoons ground chia seed (helps constipation)

½ cup chopped coriander

2 tbsp. coconut or rice bran oil

Method:

Cut the potatoes into quarters and cook for 15-25 minutes until they are soft. While the potatoes are cooking, steam the cauliflower for 15 minutes until tender.

Mash potatoes and transfer them to a large bowl.

Place the cauliflower in a food processor or blender with the salmon, chilli, lemon rind and lemon juice and process until the mixture is well combined but retains some texture.

Transfer to the bowl with the mashed potatoes and add the ground chia, shallots and coriander. Mix until really well combined. Using your hands, form small patties approximately 6 cm in diameter.

Heat a pan with a little oil and cook the patties on a low heat for 3-4 minutes on each side. Transfer to a baking tray lined with baking paper and place in the oven (160C) to keep warm.

Serve with a green salad.

Tips: For convenience you can do this with tinned fish; the best are from Forever Living and are sustainably caught, use sardines or trout. You can grill the patties instead of frying them just brush them with a little coconut oil.

7.   BROWN RICE WITH QUINOA PATTIES. Vegetarian/Vegan by Grace

Ingredients: Choose your own quantities

Brown rice, cooked with salt, oil and turmeric
Quinoa cooked with turmeric (cook like rice)
Pumpkin, preferably roasted (or oven baked or cooked) as a binder
Sunflower seeds, dry toasted on a pan
Fresh parsley, chopped finely
Cinnamon, ground
Nutmeg, ground
Salt, pepper, chilli powder
Polenta for coating
Oil for frying

Method:

Combine the ingredients in a large bowl and form patties. Soft pumpkin together with soft warm rice will bind the patties nicely. Season to your own preference. Coat in polenta and shallow fry. Serve with salad greens.

Tip: Rice crumbs with chickpea flour can be used instead of polenta.

When cooking rice, add an extra bit of water so rice is not fluffy but soft and sticky. Rinse rice before cooking but do not soak as soaking helps fluffiness, which we want to avoid here.

If you have stock, use stock instead of water for cooking rice and quinoa.

8.   WALNUT AND LENTIL TERRINE WITH ROSEMARY Vegetarian/Vegan by Grace

Ingredients: Choose your own quantities.

Walnuts, soaked, then chopped
Lentils (brown or green), cooked
Fresh rosemary leaves
Oil
Salt, pepper
Celery stalk, chopped
Tomatoes, fresh and chopped or tinned diced tomatoes to make a salsa

Method:

Combine walnuts and lentils in a large bowl. In a frying pan, heat up the oil, add rosemary and celery. Simmer for a while then add tomatoes, salt and pepper. Transfer the salsa into the bowl with lentils and mix all together. Season as preferred. Grease the terrine/loaf form and fill up with the mixture. Bake for half an hour at 180°C.

Tips: Soaked nuts are better for digestion. You can also use almonds. When you mix lentils, use firm movements so that some of the lentils break down. You can also blend half of the lentils in a food processor for better binding.

9.   HERBED ZUCCHINI AND SPINACH FRITTATA Vegetarian/Vegan

Ingredients:

250 g silken tofu
150 g firm tofu 1 small packet
1 zucchini – sliced and fried or steamed or spaghetti style using a spiraliser

1 small bunch spinach

1 tablespoon dill, fresh, chopped finely

1 tsp. thyme, fresh, chopped

Pinch black Indian salt

Pinch black pepper

Coconut oil or butter

Method:

Blend both silken and firm tofu in a food processor with black salt and dill. Transfer into a bowl. Sautee zucchini and thyme in a frying pan with coconut oil, then add spinach to it and simmer until spinach is wilted. Add warm zucchini/spinach to the bowl with tofu and mix together. Add pepper to taste. Transfer into a greased flat quiche form and bake for about 30 minutes at 160°C.

Tip: Add black salt little by little while processing the tofu and taste until you are happy with the saltiness. Black salt mimics the flavour of eggs and it pretty salty so you will not need any regular salt.

10. TEMPEH DELIGHT - Vegetarian/Vegan

Ingredients:

1 packet of tempeh, cut into very thin slices

2 cm fresh turmeric root chopped

2 cm fresh ginger root, chopped

2 garlic cloves finely chopped

1 onion finely chopped

4 tablespoons of rice bran oil or coconut oil or a mixture of both

Tamari (avoid with candida) or herb salt to taste

A selection of chopped vegetables

Method:

Add the oil to the pan. Add the tempeh strips then sprinkle with tamari or herb salt.

Add all the other ingredients and fry gently for a few minutes until the tempeh turns golden brown on one side and then turn over. Add the vegetables cook until the tempeh is golden brown on the other side. Serve with quinoa, brown rice, buckwheat, with salads or in sandwiches.

Tip: The trick to tasty tempeh is to cut it really thin, about 2mm, and cook it really well. It will then have a delicious nutty flavour. Tempeh promotes healthy intestinal flora though not advised if you have candida.

11. VEGGIE DAHL - Vegetarian/ Vegan

Ingredients:

1 cup yellow split pea mung dahl - wash well in a colander
4 cups filtered water
1 tbsp. coconut oil or ghee
1 tsp. cumin
1 tsp. grated ginger
1 tsp. mustard seeds
1 tsp. coriander ground
1 tsp. turmeric
1 onion chopped
2 cloves garlic chopped
1 cinnamon stick - remove after cooking
A pinch of chilli if desired
½ cup veggies of your choice
1 tsp. Celtic or Himalayan salt

Method:

Fry onions and garlic in coconut oil until slightly brown. Add all other ingredients and simmer on a low heat for a long period of time for extra taste - you can add water as necessary. Cook it until the dahl is creamy and split peas not detectable. For extra flavour you can add a tablespoon of whey at the end which gives a lovely flavour.

Tip: You can remove garlic and onion for a different flavour. The yellow mung beans are the quickest to cook and easier to digest than lentils. It is gentle on the gut and the spices are aromatic digestives. It is also nice with tomatoes added near the end. Adding a teaspoon of cumin and a kombu stick whilst cooking takes out the gas forming substances.

12. JAY'S NORI ROLL UPS

These can be vegan, vegetarian or with meat fish or eggs according to the fillings you desire.

Ingredients:

Nori seaweed sheets
Tamari
Cooked brown rice or another grain
Stir fried or raw vegetables: consider garlic, onion and turmeric in the mix
Protein of your choice

Method:

Mix the rice, a few sprinkles of tamari and vegetables with a protein of your choice. Place the mixture on the inner third of a nori sheet and roll up. Seal the nori with wet fingers.

Tips: Eat like a mountain bread roll up, experiment with different fillings. Chopped Umeboshi plums work well in the mix.

13. BUCKWHEAT KASHA - Vegetarian/Vegan also for meat/fish dishes

Ingredients:

1 cup buckwheat
2 ½ cups water
Pinch Celtic or Himalayan salt

Method:

Put the buckwheat into a frying pan, turn the stove on low and dry roast the buckwheat, stirring consistently until brown. Slowly add 1 cup of water to the pan and simmer until absorbed. Place the buckwheat in an oven proof dish and add the remaining 1½ cups of water and the salt. Do not cover. Bake at 180°C for 1-1½ hours until the water has absorbed and the top is brown and crunchy. Serve with salads, mains or vegetables or add berries, yoghurt or kefir and cinnamon for a healthy dessert.

Tip: Buckwheat is very helpful for haemorrhoids.

4   Sugar free desserts

Sweet foods are not recommended until you are feeling better. These are healthy sweet treats and great for birthdays, not for candida.

1.   GEORGIA'S CHOCOLATE CAKE

Ingredients:

250g coconut oil or coconut butter. Depending on the weather coconut oil can be solid or liquid. If it is solid put in a pan on a low heat until liquid; if you can tolerate butter you can use it.
4 tbsp. chia seeds soaked in a cup of water for 15 minutes
½ cup raw cocoa
5 medium eggs (If you are intolerant to eggs you can double the amount of chia seeds for more binding though the texture will be a bit different.)
1 cup almond meal
1 cup coconut palm sugar or other sweeteners like yacon syrup, rice syrup or stevia
Pinch of Celtic or Himalayan salt
1 tsp bicarbonate of soda

Method:

Whisk the eggs with a fork until they blend, then mix these with all the other ingredients in a large bowl. Place the mixture in an average sized cake tin or loaf tin and bake at 180°C for about

45 minutes. You may want to brush the tin with coconut oil or line with baking paper to make it easy to extract.

Serve warm or cold. Yummy and very moist!

Tip: This is absolutely delicious! It tastes naughty but is full of healthy ingredients and easy to make. If you are allergic to eggs also see egg replacements in Ch.11

2. BLISS CAKE

Ingredients:

Crust

2 cups walnuts
2 cups almonds
8 dates

Process in a food processor until smooth

Lemon cream

1½ cups macadamia nuts
½ cup honey, rice syrup or stevia
2 tbsp. lemon juice (if you like lime you can use it instead)
¼ cup of water

Process in a high powered food processor like Vitamix until smooth

Icing cream

2 cups coconut meat or cashew nuts
1 cup pine nuts
¼ cup honey
¼ cup coconut water

Process in a high powered food processor until smooth

4 tbsp. dried coconut powder

Fruit

You can choose what fruit you would like, thinly sliced e.g. banana, papaya and mango.

Method:

Put half of the crust into a flan base or cake tin. Push it hard until it is firm all around. Place thin slices of banana to cover the base. Put another layer of crust over the banana, push down firmly and then pour the lime cream on top. Then add slices of papaya and mango on top and pour the icing cream over that. Then add another layer of papaya and mango slices all over the top. Lastly, sprinkle dried coconut all over the last layer and put it in the fridge for an hour. It's then ready to serve.

Tip: This is raw and therefore requires no cooking. Not for those with candida. This takes a bit of time but is worth it as the taste is sensational.

3.   **SWEET INDULGENCE**

Ingredients:

1 cup coconut oil
¾ cup xylitol or stevia or rice syrup (or equivalent of ¾ cup sugar)
2 eggs
2tsp vanilla essence or the contents of 2 vanilla pods
½ cup rice flour
½ cup coconut flour
1 cup of almond meal
½ tsp. Celtic salt
½ tsp. baking powder
1 cup shredded coconut

¾ cup cocoa powder or carob powder (you may want to lessen sweetener with carob powder as it is sweet

2 crushed cardamom pods

Optional ¾ cup of grated carrots or sliced bananas or nuts or seeds

Method:

Preheat oven to 180°C. Combine coconut oil and sweeteners in a mixer until creamy then add eggs and vanilla essence. In a separate bowl mix flour, salt and baking powder and add to the other mixture, then add other ingredients. Spoon mixture onto a baking tray and bake for about 30 minutes. When cool, cut into bite size pieces.

Tips: Add ginger, fennel seeds or cinnamon for a different flavour.

4.   CAROB WALNUT BROWNIES

Ingredients:

¼ cup coconut oil

6 tbsp. carob powder

1 cup rice syrup or alternative sweetener (yacon syrup, xylitol, coconut sugar, stevia)

½ cup rice flour

½ cup coconut flour

1 cup almond meal

¼ tsp. celtic salt

2 tsp vanilla extract or vanilla pod

2 egg whites

1 cup chopped walnuts

Method:

Preheat oven to 175°C. Grease an 8 inch square baking tin with coconut oil or rice bran oil. Melt coconut oil over a low heat. Stir in other ingredients leaving egg whites and walnuts until last. Place dough evenly in baking tin. Bake for 30 minutes and cool for 15 minutes before cutting.

Tips: Carob powder is a natural sweet alternative to cocoa which, unlike cocoa, is caffeine free.

2   Breads

No breads are recommended in the initial stages of gut problems. If carbohydrates are tolerated, the best ones are brown rice, quinoa, buckwheat and millet. Commercial bread is full of preservatives, additives and yeast. Here are a couple of healthy breads which can be used as snacks with a healthy savoury dip.

1.   ZUCCHINI LOAF

Ingredients:

2 ½ cups brown rice, cooked
2 ½ cups grated zucchini
½ tsp. vegetable salt
1 tsp thyme
Pinch fennel seeds
Tbsp. dried coriander
1 chopped onion
Sesame seeds
Olive oil
3 beaten eggs

Method:

Preheat the oven to 220°C. Mix all ingredients and put into a loaf tin, brush the top with olive or coconut oil then sprinkle sesame seeds on top. Bake for 20 minutes to ½ hour.

2. CORN BREAD

Ingredients:

Preheat the oven to 220°C. You will need an 8 inch loaf tin.
1 cup rice milk or oat milk or almond milk
1 egg
1 cup yellow corn meal/polenta
1 cup buckwheat flour or rice flour
3 tbsp. melted coconut oil
2 tsp. baking powder
1 tsp baking soda
½ tsp. Celtic or Himalayan salt

Method:

Beat the egg and milk. Mix the dry stuff and combine everything in the pan. Cook for 20 minutes.

Tip: Eggs are highly nutritious however, if you are intolerant see ch. 11 for some alternatives.

For more delicious recipes go to www.detoxspecialist.com.au

CHAPTER 13

Workbook

"*The more severe the pain or illness the more severe will be the necessary changes. These may involve breaking bad habits or acquiring some new and better ones.*"

Peter Mcwilliams

CHAPTER 13
Workbook

"No time for your health today, no health for your time tomorrow."
Proverb

Changing your diet and lifestyle to achieve a better level of health can be quite daunting. Some people will take the changes on and then give up finding it all too hard, feel deprived and then go on an unhealthy binge. The key is to set yourself achievable goals that are specific, realistic, measurable and time based. For example, "On April 12th I am cutting down my coffee by two a day. I will go for a walk during work breaks and avoid the coffee machine. I will record my achievements in my diary. By 12th May I will have achieved a month of 2 fewer coffees a day and be ready to eliminate coffee altogether," or whatever the choice is for you.

You are the creator of your own unique body and you can move towards health and happiness if you aren't there yet! It's so important to take steps to make a difference to your well-being, as health is the main thing that determines happiness. Keep this in mind as you allow yourself to be strong at sticking to your goals.

Celebrate your achievements but not with food. You could spend time in nature, buy a new plant or flowers for yourself, take a weekend away or watch the sunset. Keep focus on your end goal and what you are achieving and remember happiness is a complete regular bowel motion with no discomfort, bloating, constipation or diarrhoea and you'll get there. There are weekly gifts you can give to yourself to improve your digestion and overall health. Stop telling yourself you have no time, you'll do it when you've finished the next big project, you'll wait until the kids grow up or you'll do it when your kitchen is organised.

Start now with small achievable steps towards wellness and you will reap the rewards of feeling great, feeling younger and have the vibrancy you want to do the things you love. The important thing is to keep moving forward, even if you have a relapse or binge. You can't do anything about your habits in the past but you can keep moving forward now. We all make mistakes and can learn from them, even the big mistakes.

Often if you've tried something and it hasn't worked, you are not doing it for long enough or properly. Trying to do something usually means giving up or not committing. It takes a lot more energy trying to do something rather than just doing it.

Your family and friends may think you are a little crazy for eating healthy food but when they see the changes in you they'll want what you have. You will have times where you feel like stopping and going backwards, that's human nature. Just be gentle with yourself and think of the next step you can take in a positive direction.

As you learn to nurture yourself you will move beyond your pain or discomfort and relish a new level of health. The experience is empowering when you know you can create your own good health.

How long it takes is very individual and it is worthwhile following this to feel better and give yourself a better quality of life. Health is everything and without it life is not nearly as enjoyable.

Some of you will feel fantastic in as little as three weeks and for others it may take a couple of years to reach peak health but you will feel yourself improving all the time.

So set yourself a window of time each week, to plan your food at home and discover the healthy places to eat out and the healthy juice bars.

Some of you may like to do something different every day for 100 days to create better health. This may be around food, drink, exercise, stress levels or spirituality.

Others might want to create 1 habit for 28 days before moving to the next health goal.

I'd suggest you follow what is recommended, however, if it's not realistic for you then do something that is. If you don't complete the task each week go back and spend another week on it until you've mastered a new habit or technique or changed your thinking.

SIGN THE CONTRACT!

Contract

I_____, commit myself to eight weeks of changing my diet and lifestyle habits.

I commit to implementing dietary changes and weekly tasks.

I_____ understand that this course will raise issues and emotions for me to deal with but I will keep going and work through this.

I_____ commit to my health, adequate sleep, improving my diet, exercise, sunshine, fresh air, positive friendships, doing things I love, clean filtered water and pampering.

Sign _____

Date _____

WEEK ONE

Steps towards wellness

Open up your food cupboards and take out anything that isn't a whole food from nature.

Take out anything with sugar or white flour. Look at your packets and tins; do they have additives, preservatives, colours or are they dead and denatured foods? Put anything that doesn't come from nature in the bin, they are not fit for anyone to eat.

Go to the market or health food shop and invest in healthy whole food. Buy fresh fruit and vegetables. If you need some tins of food buy them from the organic shop. Drink filtered or bottled water and get rid of any cordials, fizzy or soft drinks as they have no goodness at all.

Write a meal plan for the week so you know what food to have in the house and if you are going out, experiment with healthier foods on the menu or one less wine than normal.

WEEK TWO

Did you manage your steps towards wellness for week one?

What did you do and how did you feel?

Were there any challenges?

Is there anything you need to adjust in your life to help you stay on the wellness path?

Steps towards wellness for week two

Things to do

Make yourself a diet diary like the one below and fill in what you eat and drink for the week. Also include any exercise you do and your bowel movements each day. You will gain awareness of what you are putting into your body and how it is affecting your digestion. You can then use this diet diary each week.

	Monday	Tuesday	Wednesday	Thursday	Friday	Saturday	Sunday
Breakfast							
Lunch							
Dinner							
Snacks							
Water/ drinks							
Exercise							
Bowel movements							

List Seven little changes you would like to do for yourself to improve your health.

For example, "I would like to drink two litres of water a day."

Or "I would like to stop eating lollies." Then commit to it.

Cut your caffeine consumption in half if you drink it. If you drink alcohol have 3 alcohol free days and cut your other consumption in half.

WEEK THREE

Did you manage your steps towards wellness for week two?

What did you do and how did you feel?

Were there any challenges?

Is there anything you need to adjust in your life to help you stay on the wellness path?

Take action and implement the changes you would like to achieve after evaluating your diet sheet from week 2.

Steps towards wellness

Things to do

So how alkaline or acid are you? Get yourself some pH strips which are often sold at health food stores. Start testing your pH two hours or more after a meal, not before breakfast. Tear off a small amount of the yellow paper and wee on it and it will change colour in seconds. You ideally want your pH to be around 6.6, below that your body is getting more acidic and not absorbing minerals. If it is very high (above 7.5) your body may be too alkaline, congested and also not absorbing minerals effectively.

If you are acidic introduce more green vegetables, vegetable juices, lemons, Umeboshi plums and lower your sugar and caffeine intake.

Buy some organic lemons or get some from a friend who has a lemon tree. Lemons are highly alkaline inside the body. Squeeze a lemon a day into water; drinking it first thing and sipping it with meals is wonderful for digestion and cleansing. Lemon also helps weight loss. Remember to rinse your mouth with water after having lemon as the acid inside your mouth can affect the enamel on your teeth.

WEEK 4

Did you manage your steps towards wellness for week three?

What did you do and how did you feel?

Were there any challenges?

Is there anything you need to adjust in your life to help you stay on the wellness path?

Take action and implement the changes you would like to achieve after evaluating your diet sheet from week 3.

Steps towards wellness

Things to do

Are you using any junk food for the soul. Are you poisoning yourself with sugar or alcohol or other foods? How can you feed your soul with something positive, that will make you feel fantastic? Make some changes and trust that a stronger and clearer you is emerging.

Ideas to feed your soul: Aromatherapy baths, flowers, listen to music you love, walk in nature, eat healthy food or vegetable juice, read a good book or talk to a friend.

Be aware of poisonous friends. Health flourishes when you have a sense of safety and self-acceptance. You need to be around safe companions who support you, as toxic playmates can turn over all your good intentions. Some friends may find your recovery disturbing. Your friends, feeling neglected by your movement from unhealthy living may unconsciously try to guilt trip you into undoing new healthy habits. Be careful to safeguard yourself. Do not let them waste your time. Be gentle but firm and hang in there for what's right for you. Eventually they may learn from you. Look for new hobbies to meet new friends if you feel the need. For example, if you are with a crowd that drinks excessively this makes it hard for you to heal. You could go to healthy cooking classes or a yoga class to meet new people.

Take wheat flour and gluten out of your diet and start to include whole grains like brown rice, quinoa, buckwheat or millet. You can use these as a cereal or with any main meal. See Ch11 kitchen pharmacy and the recipes in Ch12 for ideas.

WEEK 5

Did you manage your steps towards wellness for week four?

What did you do and how did you feel?

Were there any challenges?

Is there anything you need to adjust in your life to help you stay on the wellness path?

Take action and implement the changes you would like to achieve after evaluating your diet sheet from week 4.

How can you celebrate your achievements so far?

Things to do

If you go out and you feel pressured into eating something you know isn't good for you don't worry about pleasing others, think more about valuing yourself, then you will be happier and more useful for others.

Quick quiz:

My biggest difficulty with my diet is...

What I am doing right with my diet is....

Steps I can take to improve my diet are....

One reason that I sabotage my diet is....

I can move forward by....

Am I drinking enough water?

If I were 80 I would like my health to be... and my life would look like...

WEEK 6

Did you manage your steps towards wellness for week five?

What did you do and how did you feel?

Were there any challenges?

Is there anything you need to adjust in your life to help you stay on the wellness path?

Take action and implement the changes you would like to achieve after evaluating your diet sheet from week 5.

Things to do

10 ways I can improve my diet (use tips in this book)...

10 things that are already looking better arc...

3 kitchen items I would like to own are...

The benefits of improving my diet are....

Use more kitchen herbs in your diet to aid digestion (see kitchen pharmacy). Start to add them to cooked food and experiment with making your own stocks.

WEEK 7

Did you manage your steps towards wellness for week six?

What did you do and how did you feel?

Were there any challenges?

Is there anything you need to adjust in your life to help you stay on the wellness path?

Take action and implement the changes you would like to achieve after evaluating your diet sheet from week 6.

Things to do

Leave enough time in your life to cook something that makes you happy and joyous and gives you good health.

Cook something new from the recipe section.

Clear out anything left in your cupboards that doesn't serve your health.

Incorporate a bowel exercise (from the book) daily.

Add more green leafy vegetables to your daily diet like bok choy, silverbeet, chard, rocket and kale. These have an abundance of minerals and your liver and bowel will love them.

Are you treating yourself well?

Are you enjoying wonderful kitchen smells?

Buy yourself a groovy kitchen apron.

WEEK 8

Did you manage your steps towards wellness for week seven?

What did you do and how did you feel?

Were there any challenges?

Is there anything you need to adjust in your life to help you stay on the wellness path?

Take action and implement the changes you would like to achieve after evaluating your diet sheet from week 7.

Things to Do

Have you eaten fermented food? Make yourself something fermented (see Ch.9) and have it every day for 7 days.

What action can you take now to improve your diet for the next 90 days?

Where would you like to be in a year with your health?

List 5 things you will avoid in your diet.

List 5 things you will include in your diet.

Use an enema or book in for a colonic hydrotherapy/irrigation appointment.

I allow myself...to plan my food and....time in the kitchen.

List 5 small victories you have had over the last few weeks.

Make a list of the healthy foods you love and plan meals with them.

Take an empty jar and each day write out at least 1 thing you have done towards improving your health. At the end of the year open your jar and look at all the positive steps you have made.

You are doing well. A path is emerging, insights, clarity, vitality are happening. Celebrate your success and keep it up.

For the next 90 days continue to work on your health to set habits.

List 10 ways you will continue to nurture yourself over the next 3 months.

Write out a plan for the next week: shopping, preparing, cooking and eating.

Write yourself an encouraging letter about your health and well-being. Think of how you'd write to your best friend. Then post it.

Sometimes setbacks happen; this is life, everyone has difficult days and life doesn't always go as planned. You can choose to spring back quickly as your success is not determined by your circumstance but instead by your response.

For your recovery, continue committing to your health.

New contract

I_____ am recovering and gaining vitality. To grow more in health and happiness I now commit to looking after myself for 90 days.

The last few weeks have been an important part of my recovery. I allow myself to explore healthy food and realise it is critical for good health. For the next 90 days my plan is _____
_____
_____
_____

I have chosen as support _____
and someone I can be accountable to on a weekly basis. I will start my new commitments on

_____

Sign _____

Date _____

Congratulations on your journey so far. I wish you the best health and happiness.

You are doing so well, why not continue for another 90 days!

"To keep the body in good health is a duty otherwise we shall not be able to keep our mind strong and clear."

Buddha

INDEX

Page numbers followed by c and f indicate information found in charts and figures respectively.

D

Author's Final Word

For every person who reads this book and works through the changes they need to make, it is my desire that you have been inspired and motivated to achieve a greater level of health. You can then progress towards a long, healthy, happy and productive life.

The digestive system is the cause of most health problems and I have seen the extraordinary impact diet has, both negatively and positively.

Enjoy your experiences, new choices and the journey. The ride can be rough but it always changes for the better, if you are making positive moves in the right direction.

You can do it! Start with one small change, then the next.....

Good luck

I wish you all the best for a happy tummy.

Michèle Wolff

ABOUT THE AUTHOR

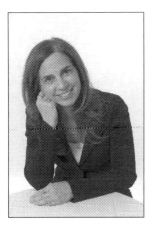

Michèle Wolff is a qualified skilled naturopath, nurse, hypnotherapist, trainer, successful business owner, highly sought after speaker, a digestive expert and an author.

Growing up in England as the eldest of seven children, Michèle developed a drive at a young age to make a difference through voluntary work and helping others less fortunate than herself, particularly those suffering serious illness.

Over the years living in different countries Michèle herself experienced serious ongoing health issues and discovered the power of natural medicine to treat and overcome her ailments. This personal experience led to a passion to study and work in the field of health.

Michèle has a Bachelor of Health Science degree in Naturopathy, and a Diploma in Nutrition and Herbal Medicine. She is qualified as a Registered Nurse, Colonic hydrotherapist, Ericksonian Hypnotherapist, Neuro Linguistic Programming practitioner and Aromatherapist. Michèle uses all of her skills - such as herbal medicine, nutrition, aromatherapy oils, massage, colonics, diet and hypnosis - to enhance digestive health.

Bringing together her studies in western and natural medicine, she treats a wide range of issues, treating each person as an individual. Michèle enjoys seeing people reach their health goals and educates people on how to live long, healthy and productive lives.

She pioneered Closed Colonics when she came to Australia from London in 1992. She also founded the Indian and Oriental Head Massage Institute and trains people to teach and perform this unique massage. She is the founder and owner of Ultimate Detox Solutions, a leading clinic using a variety of specialist treatments to take people to optimal health. Michèle is also a certified

Hypnobirthing Practitioner, running classes for pregnant mothers who want to birth in an easy and comfortable way.

She is an expert in digestive comfort and detoxifying the body naturally, for peak energy, wellness and preventing disease. Her expertise in Food as Medicine for optimal performance is often sought after by businesses, sports clubs and organisations, as well as individuals.

For over 20 years Michèle's expertise has been in high demand. She has lectured around the world for universities and private companies, spoken on radio and had articles published in magazines and newspapers. She has also organised international health related conferences.

Michèle applies her passion for Food as Medicine to her own life. She has seen first-hand both the extraordinary positive and negative impacts of diet. She is passionate about changing the way communities eat and think about food, which will lead to positive change in the food industry.

Michèle is a member of the Australian Natural Therapists Association, Australian Traditional Medicine Society and Australian Colon Health Association.

A keen artist, Michèle also enjoys cooking healthy food, the outdoors and hiking. She has visited and lived in many countries around the world, travelling both for business and pleasure.

Michèle lives in Melbourne. She visits England regularly to see her parents, six siblings and 20 cousins.

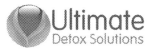

Ultimate Detox Solutions

Specialist digestive consultations, colonic irrigation, testing needs, clay, enema kits, Mg salts, zen chi machines, lymphacisers and water units

To contact the author +613 9584 7327 or info@detoxspecialist.com.au
www.detoxspecialist.com.au

RESOURCES

Soul Transformation. Experience the profound effects of this incredible consciousness technology

E=VS The Melbourne Project

+61499 106 242

www.eequalsvs.com.au

High powered blender excellent for smoothies and for many recipes

Vitamix

PO Box 158 West Wallsend NSW 2286

1800 990 990

www.vitamix.com.au

Hair Tissue Mineral Analysis for Australia and New Zealand

InterClinical Laboratories

PO Box 6474 Alexandria NSW 2015 Australia

+612 9693 2888

www.interclinical.com.au

High Quality Rice Bran Oil, available from leading health food stores and supermarkets

King Rice Bran Oil

www.ribo.com.au

+618 8354 3333

High quality Organic Food products

VICTORIA

Victoria Organic Delivery
+613 9460 3999
www.victoriaorganicdelivery.com.au

QUEENSLAND

Organic & Quality Foods
+617 3275 3552
www.organicfoods.com.au

Effective products for eliminating Geopathic Stress, Electromagnetic radiation, mobile phone, wifi and aeroplane radiation

Orgone Effects Australia
+613 9775 4122
www.orgoneffectsaustralia.com

Also available from www.detoxspecialist.com.au

High Quality Skin Brushes

Bodecare
+617 3870 0860
www.bodecare.com

Quality natural personal Lubricant

Sylk is perfect for sensitive skin and uniquely made from an extract of the kiwifruit vine. Sylk is sustainable and widely recommended.
www.sylk.com.au or phone +617 54711908

Natural Fertility Expert

Helping Hormones and Fertility Naturally
Ann Vlass
+613 9859 5629
www.helpingnatureheal.com.au

Expert Pain Management

Get a Life Integrated Health – Verona Chadwick
Author of "How to live a life without pain"
+612 6622 2436
www.getalifephysioacupuncture.com
www.howtolivealifewithoutpain.com

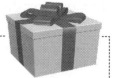

Specialists in high quality supplements in many countries

Nutrition Care Pharmaceuticals Pty Ltd
25-27 Keysborough Avenue
Keysborough VIC 3173
Australia
1800 034 445 Melbourne www.nutritioncare.com.au

Media coach for fitness and well being professionals.

Christianne Wolff
www.celebritytrainercoach.com

Natural household products, oils, teas, food, natural skin and hair care supplies.

Great Earth Health Stores

www.greatearth.com

90 Elizabeth Street, Melbourne VIC 3000 Tel: +613 9639 2533

255 Elizabeth Street, Melbourne VIC 3000 Tel: +613 9642 2788

272 Swanston Street, Melbourne VIC 3000 Tel: +613 9663 7322

Balwyn VIC Tel: +613 9888 4466

Camberwell Junction VIC Tel: +613 9882 3322

Camberwell VIC Tel: +613 9813 4888

East Doncaster VIC Tel: +613 9841 5170

For Hot Detoxifying yoga look up **Bikram Yoga** centres near you

Wholefood Chefs

MELBOURNE

Sue Stotts,

Cooking classes

www.suddenlyslender.com.au

ADELAIDE

Grace Love,

Bliss Organic Cafe

7 Compton Street, Adelaide SA 5000 (just off Gouger Street)

+618 8231 0205

www.blissorganiccafe.com

Books

Arabella Forge (2010) Frugavore: How to grow your own, buy local, waste nothing and eat well. Black Inc, Australia

Eve Hillary (1997) Children of a Toxic Harvest: An Environmental Biography. Lothian Books, Australia

Nicole Bijlsma (2012) Healthy Home, Healthy Family. Joshua books, Australia.

Rachel Carson (1962) Silent Spring. Riverside Press, Cambridge; MA Riverside.

Rick Smith, Bruce Lourie (2009), Slow Death by Rubber Duck: How the Toxic Chemistry of Everyday Life Affects our Health. University of Queensland Press, Australia.

Sarah Lantz (2009) Free kids: Raising Healthy Children in a Toxic World. Joshua books, Australia.

Sandra Steingraber (2001) Having Faith: An Ecologist's Journey to Motherhood. Berkley Publishing, U.S.A.

Stacey Malkan (2007) Not Just a Pretty Face: The Ugly Side of the Beauty Industry. New Society Publishers, Canada.

Theo Colburn, Dianne Dumanoski, John Peterson-Myers (1996). Our Stolen Future: Why Are We Threatening Our Fertility, Intelligence and Survival? Penguin Books, New York. http:/www. ourstolenfuture.org

Verona Chadwick (2012) How to live a life without pain. Global publishing, Australia www. howtolivealifewithoutpain.com

Films

The Future of Food

Food Matters

Food Inc.

Simply Raw

Reports and Journal Articles

Landrigan, P. Carlson, J. Bearer, C. et al. (1998) Children's Health and the Environment: A New Agenda for Prevention Research, Environmental Health Perspective, 1998 June; 106 (3) pp. 784-794.

Online Chemical Databases

To discover if the products you are using have harmful chemicals in them:

Environmental Working Group's Skin Deep Database www.cosmeticsdatabase.com

Safety Information Resources Database - Material Safety Data Sheet www.hazard.com/msds

ONE Group Chemical Ingredients Directory www.heathylife.Mionegroup.com/toxic

Bill Statham's The Chemical Maze www.possibiliy.com.au

Popular books you can download by Jo Imming on toxicity www.joimmig.com

Online resources Australia

Australia's National Toxics Network www.ntn.org.au on environmental health issues.

Safer Solutions: Keeping Your Home Healthy and Green www.safersolutions.org.au From this you can download a free copy of the booklet Detox Your Home.

The National Research Centre for Environmental Toxicology - Post Grad Research Centre at Queensland University www.entox.uq.edu.au

National Pollutants Inventory Database www.npi.gov.au This shows per postcode toxic emissions in Australia and where they come from.

Fluoride Action Network www.fluoridealert.org Education on the dangers of fluoride.

Australian Breastfeeding Association www.breastfeeding.asn.au

Alcohol and breastfeeding www.breatfeeding.asn.au/bfino/ABA_Alcholol_BF.pdf

Genetically modified food information www.truefood.org.au

Online resources - International

Cultured food www.culturedfoodlife.com

Ferments www.fermentersclub.com

Environmental Working Group (EWG) www.ewg.orgwww.ewg.org/kidsafewww.ewg.org/kid-safe-chemicals-act-10-americans-video Excellent reports on contaminants that affect children, pregnant mothers and pets.

The Environmental Working Group's 10 Americans Video www.ewg.org/health-Tipswww.ewg.org/reprts/body/burden2/contentindex.php

Campaign for Safe Cosmetics to eliminate links to cancer and birth defects www.safecosmetics. orgwww.safecosmetics.orgwww.cosmeticdatabase.org

Silent Spring Institute www.silentspring.orgwww.silentspring.org?sciencereview Articles on breast cancer and the environment. It provides a database on 216 chemicals shown to cause mammary gland cancer in animals.

RobertGammal.com. Dangers of root canals.

The Stockholm Convention on Persistent Organic Pollutants http://chm.pops.int 164 Nations involved in phasing out chemicals that affect its citizens.

International POP's Elimination Network www.ipen.org Government organisations working on eliminating pollutants.

Natural resources Defence Council www.nrdc.org/breatmilk Green living and contaminants in breast milk.

Crinnion Medical www.crinnionmedical.com Practical solutions to help you identify toxins in your life and how to clear them.

www.westonaprice.org. Nutrient dense food, diet and agriculture.

Robert Gamma lwww.robertgammal.com A dentist campaigning against mercury and fluoride.

Metametrix Institute - Clinical Laboratory www.metametrix.com/toxins www.diagnosticinsight. com.au Clinical laboratory tests that identify toxins underlying chronic disease and nutrient imbalances. A variety of tests that reveal a person's toxic burden.

BIBLIOGRAPHY

Abdeen, K. "Kirans whole food," recipe contributor Mornington

Astuti, M., et al. 2000 'Tempeh, a nutritious and healthy food from Indonesia'. Asia Pacific Journal of Clinical Nutrition. 9 (4). 322-325

Australian Consumers Association 2000, *How safe is our food?:* Random house Australia

Australian Organic Journal Autumn 2003. P43

Barzel U.S and Massey 1998, 'Excess dietary protein can adversely affect bone density' L.K Journal of Nutrition., Vol 6, pp, 1051-1053

Brown, S 1996, *Better Bones, Better Body,* Keats Publishing Inc.

Bobby L et al. 2010, *Trade and consumer protection,* United States House of Representatives, Washington D.C. 20515, Chemicals in umbilical cord

Cameron, J 1995,. *The Artists Way* Pan Books

Campaign for food safety issue 200 consumer report

Colbin, A 1986. *Food and Healing,* Ballantine

Collings, J1996. *Principles of Colonic Irrigation,* Thorsons

Cousens, G2000. *Conscious Eating,* Berkeley, North Atlantic Books

Dawber, Thomas et al. 1948-1966. 'The Framingham Study'

Dobbyn, S 2008, *The Fertility Diet,* Simon and Schuster

E numbers at ChemBase.com

Edwards, P, Sir, Prof 2003, *Happiness Is A Regular Complete Bowel Motion,* Pan Harmony International

Environmental working group 2006, *Dioxin in Umbilical cords,* The National Academy of Sciences,

Erasmus, U 1993., *Fats that heal Fats that Kill,* Alive Books

Fallon, S2001, *Nourishing Traditions,* New Trends Publishing

Fisher, L1993, *The Clinical Science of Mineral Therapy,* The Maurice Blackmore Research Foundation

Gates, D 2006. *The Body Ecology Diet,* B.E.D. Publications U.S.A. ninth edition

Gillard, G 2011, Anti-Ageing and the Endocrine System Seminar,

Hass, E. M 1992, *Staying Healthy with Nutrition,* Celestial Arts, California

Hu et al. 1993, 'Dietary intakes and urinary excretion of calcium and acids: a cross sectioned study of women in China', American Journal of clinical nutrition Vol 58, pp 14-19,

Isabirye-Basuta G. (1989) 'Feeding ecology of chimpanzees in the Kibale Forest, Uganda' In: Heltne PG, Marquardt LA, editors. Understanding chimpanzees. Cambridge, (MS): Harvard UnivPr; p 116-27

Healthworld 2007, *Key clinical concepts in immunology*

Whitten, KW et al. 2009 *Chemistry,* 9th Edition, Cengage Learning

Koeman, M 2012. *Stress and Fatigue, A mental health issue,* seminar by Flordis

Lee, W & Wunderlich R 1991, *The Friendly Bacteria,* Contemporary Publishing Group, Lincolnwood USA

Licata et al. 1981, 'Acute effects of dietary protein on calcium metabolism in patients with osteoporosis', Journal of gerontology. Volume 36. pp 14-19, 1981

Lomman, D2007: *RBTI Analysis Manual*

Love, G, recipe contributor, *Confident Cooking*

Manocha, Dr. R 2012, *Meditation Research Programme*, Sydney University

McCann, et al. 2007, 'Food additives and hyperactive behaviour in 3-year-old and 8/9-year-old children in the community: a randomised, double-blinded, placebo-controlled trial.' Lancet, 370: 1560–67

Mediherb 2010, *Whole life vitality detox for health program manual*

Mulder, J 2011, *The complete Ayurvedic cookbook,* 4th edition

Minakshi, D, et al. 1999, 'Antimicrobial screening of some Indian spices.' Phytotherapy research. 13 (7) 616-618

National Institute of diabetes and digestive and kidney diseases - Your digestion and how it works, viewed 20th July 2012 digestive.niddk.nih.gov/diseases/pubs/yrdd

Ohara. M., et al. 2001, 'Radioactive effects of miso against radiation in B6C3F1 mice. Increased small intestinal crypt survival, crypt lengths and prolongation of average time to death'. Hiroshima J Med Sci. 50 (4):83-86

Pitchford, P1993, *Healing with Whole Foods,* North Atlantic Books

Reddy ST et al. 2002, 'Effect of low carbohydrate high protein diets on acid-base balance, stone forming propensity and calcium metabolism'. AMJ Kidney Dis 2002;40 (2) 265-74

Sait, G2007, *Fatty Acid Fallacies and The Art of Detox,* Nutri Tech Solutions, Queensland:

Vanaitalle TB 2002, 'Stress: A risk factor for serious illness',. Metabolism 51(6) Suppl 1:40-45

Thatte.U. et al. 2000, 'Modulation of programmed cell death by medicinal plants'. Cell Mol Biol. 46. 199-214

Thomas, David. 2003, 'A study on the mineral depletion of the foods available to us as a nation over the period 1940 to 1991', Nutrition and Health, 17(2)85-115

Tucker et al. 1999 'Potassium, magnesium, and fruit and vegetable intakes are associated with greater bone mineral density in elderly men and women', American journal of clinical Nutrition Vol 69, pp727-736,

USDA 2013, *Fermented Foods,* United States Department of Agriculture, viewed 26 March 2013, www.usda.gov

Wholesomeness of food irradiated with does above 10KGy, who, Geneva 1999, Technical report series No 890

Wilcox BJ et al. 2000, Okinawan program, How the world's longest lived people achieve everlasting health Carbon/potter Pub New York

Young, O Ph.D.(& Shelley Young) 2002, The pH miracle: Warner Books

Printed in the United States
By Bookmasters